Cuba's Gay Revolution

Lexington Studies on Cuba

Series Editor

John M. Kirk, Dalhousie University, and Mervyn Bain, The University of Aberdeen

This series will publish texts on all aspects of Cuba, focusing on the post-1959 period. It seeks to be truly interdisciplinary, with studies of all aspects of contemporary Cuba—from foreign policy to culture, sociology, to economics. The series is particularly interested in broad comprehensive topics (such as women in Cuba, economic challenges, human rights, the role of the media, etc.). All ideological positions are welcomed, with solid academic quality being the defining criterion. In exceptional circumstances edited collections will be considered, but the main focus is on high quality, original, and provocative monographs and innovative scholarship.

Titles in the Series

Cuba's Gay Revolution: Normalizing Sexual Diversity Through a Health-Based Approach, by Emily J. Kirk

Cuba's Gay Revolution

Normalizing Sexual Diversity Through a Health-Based Approach

Emily J. Kirk

LEXINGTON BOOKS
Lanham • Boulder • New York • London

Published by Lexington Books
An imprint of The Rowman & Littlefield Publishing Group, Inc.
4501 Forbes Boulevard, Suite 200, Lanham, Maryland 20706
www.rowman.com

Unit A, Whitacre Mews, 26-34 Stannary Street, London SE11 4AB

British Library Cataloguing in Publication Information Available

Library of Congress Cataloging-in-Publication Data

Names: Kirk, Emily J., author.
Title: Cuba's gay revolution : normalizing sexual diversity through a health-based approach / Emily J. Kirk.
Description: Lanham : Lexington Books, [2017] | Series: Lexington studies on Cuba | Includes bibliographical references and index.
Identifiers: LCCN 2017026088 (print) | LCCN 2017030607 (ebook) | ISBN 9781498557672 (Electronic) | ISBN 9781498557665 (cloth : alk. paper)
Subjects: LCSH: Sexual minorities--Cuba. | Medical care--Cuba. | Sex instruction--Cuba,
Classification: LCC HQ73.3.C83 (ebook) | LCC HQ73.3.C83 K57 2017 (print) | DDC 306.76097291--dc23
LC record available at https://lccn.loc.gov/2017026088

∞™ The paper used in this publication meets the minimum requirements of American National Standard for Information Sciences Permanence of Paper for Printed Library Materials, ANSI/NISO Z39.48-1992.

Printed in the United States of America

This book is dedicated to John and Margo Kirk
and Yvonne and David Childs.
Thank you for everything.

Contents

Acknowledgments

Above all, I would like to thank Tony Kapcia, who has been invaluable throughout this process.

I would also like to thank CENESEX and its wonderful and dedicated staff. It has been a great honor working with a Center that undertakes such important work. Thank you for allowing me the opportunity to study your remarkable efforts and for helping me throughout the process. The dedication, compassion, creativity, and intelligence that the Center employs in its many valuable areas of work are exceptional. In particular I would like to thank Mariela Castro Espín, Ramón Rivero Pino, Yasmany Díaz Figueroa, Rosa Mayra Rodríguez Lauzurique, Manuel Vázquez Seijido, Ana María Cano López, Alberto Roque Guerra, Ada Alfonso Rodríguez, Marta María Ramírez, Pedro Pablo Valle Artiz, as well as the FMC's Carolina Aguilar Ayerra.

In addition, I would like to acknowledge Isabel Story, whose work in translation was instrumental.

I would also like to thank the extraordinary people who helped me, in various ways, and without whom this book could not have been done. Thank you Lisa Clements-Titcombe; Dennis Titcombe; Michael Kirk; Leslie Ribeiro; Doug and Noni MacDonald; Ewen and Alison MacDonald; Maartje and Gerhard Stroink; Christopher Childs; Simon Childs; Ged Santos; Nuria Díaz Varela; Jeff Scott; Hilda Power; Anne Rose; Juanita Montalvo; Magda Gonzalez-Mora; Debra Wilson; Heather Dyment; Hal Klepak; Leonardo Padura Fuentes; Sandra Ramírez; Esperanza Luzpert; Giovanni Bartolacci; Marcia, Annabel, and Frank Martínez López; Marguerite Rose Jiménez; Benjamin and Suzanne Kelly; Carlos Garduño; Chris Walker; Matthew MacLellan; Nate Pace; Laurence Brown; David Smith; Anna Clayfield; Hugo Ferreira; Raquel Ribeiro; Par Kumaraswami; Kate Ervine; Gavin Fridell; Bob Huish; Cristina Ráfeles; Stephen Roberts; Mervyn Bain; Imti Choonara; Sheryl Lutjens; Alberto Roque Guerra; Camilo Garcia López-Trigo. And a special thank you to my partner, Grant Brown.

List of Acronyms

CC: Central Committee of the Cuban Communist Party (Comité Central)
CENESEX: National Center for Sexual Education (Centro Nacional de Educación Sexual)
CDR: Committees for the Defense of the Revolution (Comité de Defensa de la Revolución)
CLASES: Latin American Congress of Sexology and Sexual Education (Congreso Latinoamericano de Sexología y Educación Sexual)
CTC: Workers Central Union of Cuba (Central de Trabajadores de Cuba)
DC: Civil Defense (Defensa Civil)
ELAM: Latin American School of Medicine (Escuela Latinoamericana de Medicina)
FEU: Federation of University Students (Federación Estudiantil Universitaria)
FMC: Federation of Cuban Women (Federación de Mujeres Cubanas)
GFATM: Global Fund to Fight AIDS, Tuberculosis and Malaria
GNTES: National Group for Work on Sexual Education (Grupo Nacional de Trabajo de Educación Sexual)
ICAIC: Cuban Institute of Cinematographic Arts and Industry (Instituto Cubano del Arte e Industria Cinematográficos)
INDER: National Institute of Sport, Physical Education and Recreation (Instituto Cubano de Deporte, Educación Física y la Recreación)
IMF: International Monetary Fund
IPPF: International Family Planning Plan (Programa Internacional de Planificación Familiar)
MINCULT: Ministry of Culture (Ministerio de Cultura)
MINJUS: Ministry of Justice (Ministerio de Justicia)
MINSAP: Ministry of Public Health (Ministerio de Salud Pública)
NSAP: National Service to Eradicate Malaria (Servicio Nacional de Erradicación de la Malaria)
OCIC: International Catholic Organization for Cinema (Organización Católica de Cine)
PCC: Cuba Communist Party (Partido Comunista de Cuba)
ProNes: National Sexual Education Programme (Programa Nacional de Educación Sexual)
ProNess: National Sexual Education and Sexual Health Program (Programa Nacional de Educación y Salud Sexual)
SAP: Structural Adjustment Program

SOCUMES: Cuba Multidisciplinary Society for the Study of Sexuality (Sociedad Cubana Multidisciplinaria para el Estudio de la Sexualidad)
UJC: Young Communist League (Unión de Jóvenes Comunistas)
UMAP: Military Aid for Production (Unidades Militares de Ayuda a la Producción)
UNDP: United Nations Development Program
UNEAC: Writers and Artists Union of Cuba (Unión de Escritores y Artistas de Cuba)
UNFPA: United Nations Family Planning Association (Fondo de Población de las Naciones Unidas)
UNIFEM: United Nations Development Fund for Women
UNJC: National Union of Cuban Jurists (Unión Nacional de Juristas de Cuba)
RSMS: Rural Social Medical Service
WHO: World Health Organization

Preface

It is perhaps pertinent to explain how this research project came about. I became interested in CENESEX during a research trip in 2008 when I was working on an earlier research project dealing with HIV/AIDS treatment and prevention strategies. Medical professionals with whom I was working, as well as members of the general population, often mentioned the Center's name and various projects it was working on, but published data on its specific role could not be found. Before leaving, I was invited by a colleague to have dinner, where serendipitously one of the Center's leading medical specialists was also in attendance. After inquiring about CENESEX and its role, the Center's significance became clear.

After two years of discussions, I was given permission from the Cuban government to conduct research at the Center and study the normalization of sexual diversity in Cuba. Following initial visits, the majority of the research was conducted over a three-month period spent at the Center and working with its faculty and staff. This book is the first time that information collected directly from CENESEX, including interviews, archival data, and observations, will be presented and their relevance discussed.

Introduction

A New Look at an Old Topic

Revolutionary Cuba has often been the focus of international news headlines. From its relationship with the United States, economic developments, visits from the Pope, work in medical internationalism, and the life of former president Fidel Castro, the Caribbean island has been the center of significant international media attention. Since 2008, however, a new story has caught the attention of international media outlets, a story on which many have reported, but few have understood—the normalization of sexual diversity in Cuba.

International reports from across North America, Latin America, the Caribbean, Europe, Asia, and Australia have discussed Cuba's work in sexual diversity rights.[1] These reports have been almost exclusively positive, lauding the country for developing new and more inclusive legislation, and hosting large-scale celebrations for the International Day Against Homophobia. They have celebrated the government's progressive attitudes toward the promotion of respect for sexual diversity, and even presented the island as something of an international leader in the normalization of sexual diversity. In particular, the National Center of Sexual Education (CENESEX), headed by Mariela Castro Espín, has routinely been noted as being at the forefront of change. For example, the *Daily Mail* reported that CENESEX "runs anti-homophobia campaigns and is lobbying for same-sex marriage to be legalized in Cuba" (*Daily Mail* 2011). Similarly, *The Advocate* reported, "[Mariela] Castro, a sexologist and director of the Cuban National Center for Sex Education (CENESEX), has long been an activist for LGBT equality in Cuba. She has been credited with improving conditions for gay Cubans, who faced imprisonment as recently as the 1970s" (Ring 2013).

These reports are more readily understood when placed in an historical context. Despite much of the positive media attention on the normalization of sexual diversity, the country has had a history of prejudice, discrimination, and violence against homosexuals. In the early years of the Revolution, many homosexual men were required to attend labor camps to help them develop a "manlier disposition" and inculcate in them revolutionary values. Legislation also institutionalized homophobia, and in effect greatly limited the lives of perceived homosexuals. Lesbians, by contrast, were largely ignored, and considered instead to be confused women who needed more guidance. Material distributed by the government across the island also strongly condemned homosexuality, describing it as an illness that could infect others, particularly young people. Homosexuality was viewed as anathema to the Revolution.

Many of the revolutionary leaders, such as Fidel Castro and Ernesto "Che" Guevara, were also notably prejudicial against homosexuals. Guevara, for example, was reported to have referred to famed homosexual Cuban writer, Reinaldo Arenas, as a "foul faggot" (Quiroga 2000, 104), while Fidel Castro noted that a homosexual could never be a true revolutionary (Lockwood 1967, 107). It was clear that for decades a state of institutionalized homophobia existed, which left its mark on sexual minorities.

These attitudes were clearly a feature of the early years of the Revolution and have continued to various degrees over the decades. As recently as 2010, Cuban delegates voted in a UN meeting to change the wording on a document that focused on discrimination, a decision that in effect supported a more homophobic agenda (Acosta 2010c). There have also been considerable debates over the 2013 Labor Code, which many have felt did not sufficiently represent sectors of the island's workforce with diverse sexual orientations, and data have also suggested that hate crimes against sexually diverse groups have actually increased. In general, however, the evidence demonstrates that discrimination by the state and general population changed significantly in 2008, when a more respectful approach began to emerge.

Since Raúl Castro was elected in 2008, attitudes toward sexual diversity have formally changed significantly. Rights, specifically, have evolved considerably, the International Day Against Homophobia has been widely celebrated, and gay film festivals have been held. The island has participated in the "Gay Olympics" and its education and medical systems have incorporated recognition and awareness of sexual diversity. Therefore, it is clear that attitudes toward sexual diversity have undoubtedly changed since the 1960s. However, for most countries this has also been the case, suggesting that Cuba is not unique is this regard. Nonetheless, the approach that was employed to normalize sexual diversity was, and remains, uniquely revolutionary and unexplored. The importance is not *what* happened, but rather *how* it happened.

Notably, many western countries have employed a rights-based approach to achieve sexual diversity rights (Ball 2010; Ibrahim 2015; Corrales 2012; Browne and Nash 2014). In Canada and the United States, for example, activist and politicians alike have demanded change based on their interpretation of human rights, citing, as an example, that it was a human rights violation not to allow homosexuals to marry (Ball 2010; La Rose 2016). This has been a common argument in many countries to establish and protect sexual diversity rights. In Cuba, however, a very different—and particularly Cuban—approach was used. Change did not occur through a rights-based approach, but instead through a health-based approach, including the discrimination-health link. Indeed, the central theme throughout the normalization process was that of health. As Mariela Castro Espín explained, "In essence, our view is that any kind of prejudice or discrimination is damaging to health" (Reed 2006).

This book will therefore examine and analyze the normalization of sexual diversity in revolutionary Cuba. The aim is to provide a more comprehensive study of the development of attitudes toward sexual diversity—from the island's homophobic past to the significant changes that have occurred in recent decades, and specifically the development of the island's particular healthcare strategy.

It should be noted from the outset that this is not specifically a study within Gender Theory. While some of the themes and vocabulary touch on areas within the broader field of Gender and Sexuality Studies, the focus on this study is to contribute to a new understanding of the role of CENESEX and the normalization of sexual diversity in Cuba.

The "negotiative process" framework is valuable in illuminating this topic. This theory maintains that the Cuban Revolution is a complex process of negotiation that continually adapts to challenges and continues to evolve, rather than functioning as a closed political structure (Kapcia 2008; 2016). As Kapcia (2014) explains, instead of employing a strictly top-down approach, the Revolution must be understood as continually adapting, evolving and utilizing the population to debate and address problems, as well as implement solutions. This is evident, for example, throughout the varying roles of the mass organizations, such as the Committees for the Defense of the Revolution (CDRs), the Federation of Cuban Women (FMC) and the Federation of University Students (FEU), the diverse roles of the Ministries, as well as decisions made within the National Assembly. In regards to the normalization of sexual diversity, this approach is particularly useful as it allows for analysis of the evolutionary process within Cuba's unique revolutionary framework.

Indeed, while frequently understood as simply a dictatorial leadership and thus a closed political structure, in fact it is much for complex. A key component to this has been what is referred to in Cuba as the "national debate." National debate, or public debate, in this context does not refer to a formal structure of debate, but rather refers to Cuba's informal structure whereby discussions of a given topic are nation-wide and present throughout various levels of society. This can include, for example, discussions between friends and neighbours, meetings of the mass organizations, within the Ministries, the Cuban Communist Party (PCC) and throughout the National Assembly. The centralized structure of the government (single-party and socialist) has also meant that the decisions of these debates can be implemented nation-wide, equally, and with little formal opposition.

Because the story of the evolution of attitudes toward sexual diversity in Cuba has been recorded incompletely and often misunderstood, a new understanding of an old topic is required. In this context, the questions needed to be asked: how did attitudes toward sexual diversity evolve in Cuba? And what does this evolutionary process tell us about the Revolution?

In order to answer these questions, over the course of four years and three research trips, the methodology for this study consisted primarily of archival and interview-based research [see Appendix A for complete list of interviews]. The extensive archival research was mainly conducted in Cuba at the National Center of Sexual Education, the José Martí National Library, and the University of Havana's library. In particular, CENESEX's archive was examined in depth, which included training manuals, reports, journals, and books. In order to further contextualize and illuminate the normalization process, popular magazines and newspapers in Cuba from 1961–2015, such as *Mujeres*, *Bohemia*, and *Granma*, were examined. In addition, official Ministry and PCC policies, as well as the Cuban Constitution and legislation, including various Codes, were analyzed. Interview-based research was conducted with several specialists familiar with the history of the normalization process. This included FMC and *Mujeres* founder, Carolina Aguilar Ayerra; CENESEX Director, Mariela Castro Espín; as well many professionals working at CENESEX. These interviews were instructive in order to develop a fuller understanding of the archival data and its significance, as well as to provide clarification and insight. They offered essential information for the overall understanding of their respective specialties as well as the process.

Although "LGBT" (or "LGBTQ," "LGBTI," "LGBTQIAA," etc.)[2] is commonly used to discuss lesbian, gay, bisexual, or transgender people or communities, this book will instead use the term "sexual diversity." In Cuba, while the term "LGBT" is used at times, albeit rarely, this research found that "sexual diversity" was clearly the predominant terminology employed to refer to varying sexual orientations, preferences, and gender identities. The term can best be understood as somewhat of an amorphous concept that includes all diverse sexual orientations as well as gender identities. This term is used in Cuba, rather than LGBT(QIAA) because it is understood to be more inclusive of the many and varying sexual orientations, preferences, and gender identities—rather than simply categorizing or identifying specific independent sub-groups outside of heterosexual behavior. In addition, it is believed that by using one umbrella term there will be less division between the groups (namely, lesbians, gays, bisexual, and transgender persons), and will thus create, or seek to create, a united front against discrimination and prejudice. Sexual diversity as a term and concept, although not present in literature outside of Cuba, has been essential to the overall process of normalization within the island.

Moreover, similar to the Leiner's (1994) study on homosexuality in Cuba, this study will also discuss changes in "attitudes." While attitudinal change does not necessarily lend itself well to rigorous quantitative analysis, it can more broadly be understood as the general positions held within a community or country toward a given topic. Evidence for attitudes toward a theme can be extrapolated or interpreted from cultural expressions, such as popular books, official documents or statements, educational practices, and health policies. This study will employ the term to refer to the general understanding of sexual diversity, as evidenced by analysis of the archival and interview-based research conducted.

Some notable academic studies have been published on the evolution of attitudes toward sexual diversity in Cuba, with the majority appearing in the early and mid-1990s. These include the studies of Marvin Leiner (1994) and Ian Lumsden (1996), as well as research conducted by Lourdes Arguelles and Ruby B. Rich (1984; 1985), and Brad Epps (1995). Emilio Bejel (2001) has also offered some insight by examining the evolution through literature and the idea of nationhood. A recent ethnographic study has also been produced by Noelle Stout (2014), as well as a book published by Carrie Hamilton (2012) that focuses on oral history. Yet despite the voluminous amounts of media reports on the evolution of contemporary Cuba's attention to sexual diversity, as well as some important academic studies on the evolution of this process, some significant problems with the work that has been produced are apparent. In particular, noticeably little has been published since the mid-1990s. While the work of Leiner (1994) provided considerable insight into the evolutionary process and some excellent data from that period, since then there has been no work produced of similar quality. The necessary data and analysis to understand the contemporary events, as well as to provide a more comprehensive examination of the normalization process of sexual diversity, have been lacking since his initial study.

Moreover, an ongoing issue that extends throughout all published work is that a significant level of repetition is apparent, as the recent sources all propose a similar understanding of the shift in attitudes. They trace perceived major events or episodes in revolutionary Cuban history that are believed to have changed, or contributed to the change, in sexual diversity rights. These include, for example, the Military Units to Aid Production (UMAP) camps, the decriminalization of homosexuality in 1979, the 1993 release of the film *Strawberry and Chocolate* (*Fresa y Chocolate*), and finally in 2008, when Castro Espín indicated that comprehensive sexual diversity rights for all were to be her main objective as well as that of CENESEX. These are the central threads that run through the more recent texts on the broad question of sexual diversity in Cuba. While on the surface this chronology of significant isolated events is helpful in terms of understanding how much attitudes have changed, in fact it ignores what is certainly the most important component of the overall analysis, namely that the most significant contributing factor to the normalization process is CENESEX. The Center has never been studied in any real depth, and the only academic work on it and its role was published by the Center's own director, Castro Espín (2011), a Cuban physician and sexual diversity advocate, Roque Guerra (2011), as well as two other publications (Kirk 2011; 2015). This lack of information on CENESEX is mainly due to the fact that, until now, no foreign researcher has received permission to analyze the Center from within. This is largely the result of the sensitive nature of the information, as well as the Center's national prestige.

The first chapter of this book gives a comprehensive overview of revolutionary Cuba's problematic approach to homophobia until the 1990s. Following this, the subsequent chapter analyzes the establishment and early development of sexual education and sexual health programs, with an emphasis on the role of the FMC from 1959 to 1989. It explores the way in which sexual education and sexual health engaged with attitudes toward sexual diversity, as well as the establishment of the discrimination-health link. The third chapter builds on the second, following the trend of sexual education and sexual health through the development and fundamental structure of CENESEX, as well as its role in Cuba from 1989. The fourth chapter revisits the normalization of sexual diversity, examining the developments from 1990, with an emphasis on more contemporary issues. The final chapter does not focus on sexual diversity as such, but instead analyzes Cuba's approach to healthcare, in an effort to provide a greater understanding of the island's particular view of health, as the context within which CENESEX and the normalization process should be examined.

This is therefore the first comprehensive analysis of the normalization of sexual diversity in revolutionary Cuba, incorporating data that until now has never been seen outside the island. The island has responded to sexual diversity in a unique way—using particular Cuban problems and solutions to develop strategies and implement change. It is certainly a story worth telling.

NOTES

1. See, for example, Acosta 2011a; *AllAfrica.com* 2012; *Ansa Latina Roma* 2011; *BBC* 2013; *Correo del Orinoco* 2013; *Ecodiario* 2012; *El Universo* 2012; *IPS* 2012a; *La República* 2012; *San Francisco Chronicle* 2012; *Swissinfo* 2010; *Sydney Morning Herald* 2012; *Terra Perú* 2011.

2. See, for example, Goldberg et al. 2012; Guarnero and Flaskerud 2014; Sahar 2012.

ONE

Red Gays

Attitudes Toward Sexual Diversity in Cuba, 1959–1989

In a famous lecture on the topic of homosexuality in 1889, G. Frank Lydston discussed his observations on homosexuals and their behavior. He posited that groups of homosexuals existed in communities of any size, and could be easily discovered due to their "effeminacy of voice, dress, and manner." He also concluded "They are usually known to each other, and are likely to congregate together. At times they operate in accordance with some definite and concerted plan in quest of subjects wherein to gratify their abnormal sexual impulses" (Fone 2000, 347). Indeed, many societies have struggled with accepting or understanding homosexuality. In this regard, revolutionary Cuba has not been the exception.

Like many aspects of revolutionary Cuba, the evolution of attitudes toward sexual diversity is complex and controversial, and has developed since the realization of the Revolution in 1959. Almost immediately following the rebellion, myriad reports surfaced suggesting the severe repression and discrimination of homosexuals on the island.

The reasons behind the markedly negative attitudes toward sexual diversity—particularly in the 1960s and 1970s—were complex. The rooted homophobia resulted from a conflict between the cultural and economic effects of Spanish colonial rule and the United States' neocolonial rule, followed by struggles within Cuba between various external and internal forces. In revolutionary Cuba, homosexual men were often seen as being synonymous with prostitution, decadence, mental illness, and immorality. Cuban *machismo* and socially dictated gender roles would also aggravate this societal construct, as men were expected to be strong, virile, and in particular sexually dominant over women. Homosexual men, particularly effeminate ones, did not fit into the concept of *machismo*, further alienating them from much of the general populace that actively believed in, and engaged with, the development of a new Cuban society.

At the beginning of the Revolution, the leadership sought to develop a "New Man," one that espoused the essential characteristics that a true revolutionary should have—such as being honorable and morally incorruptible. In essence, the aim was to develop a truly revolutionary populace. Yet a main effect of this aim, and the means in which the government carried out this goal, resulted in an intensification of the existing homophobia. The sexually diverse, and in particular effeminate homosexual men, became the political "other," and therefore a significant problem for the Revolution.

The results of the increase in prejudice and discrimination against homosexuality included, among others, forced participation in the UMAP camps; the establishment of schools designed to change effeminate boys into masculine men; legislation barring homosexuals from various job sectors (and in particular teaching and medical appointments) for fear that they may "infect" others, as well as the criminalization of homosexual behavior. Homophobia was most prevalent throughout the 1960s and 1970s. While some changes occurred in the late 1970s and 1980s, obvious discrimination against homosexuality continued.

This chapter will outline the development of attitudes, policies, and rights toward sexual diversity, between 1959 and 1989, examining the evolution of negative attitudes and the beginning of the normalization process. While these negative attitudes toward homosexuality have typically been attributed to *machismo*, the challenge in understanding this evolutionary process is significantly more complicated, involving aspects of pre-revolutionary and revolutionary history.

SEXUAL DIVERSITY IN PRE-REVOLUTIONARY CUBA

In order to understand homophobia in revolutionary Cuba, it is instructive to first examine attitudes toward sexuality leading up to the Revolution. These attitudes were the product of almost four centuries of Spanish colonial rule, followed by the United States' neo-colonial rule. Indeed, as Brad Epps (1995, 236) noted, "The significance of homosexuality in revolutionary Cuba is the product of history." To understand sexuality during Spanish colonial rule, there are three components that must be considered: 1) *Machismo*; 2) the role of women in society; and 3) the effects of the United States' neo-colonial rule.

Machismo was a significant contributor to the Cuban populace's rejection of homosexuality, and was in many ways the result of Spanish colonial rule. However, the term has often been misunderstood, or confused with patriarchy. Although the two are linked—*machismo* is derived directly from patriarchal structures—they are also distinct. *Machismo* denotes conformity, or a performance of conformity, to dominant masculine norms (Formental Hernández et al. 2014; Baron 2011; Hirai et al. 2014; Mirandé 1997). Without patriarchy, and resulting masculine hegemony, such conformity would be meaningless (Basham 1976). However hegemonic masculinity has been reproduced at various stages throughout Latin American and Caribbean history (Firestone 1970; Seidler 1989; Dunphy 2000; Whitehead 2002; Figes 1970; Coward 1983). For example, the notion of manliness (often referred to as *hombría*) was central to indigenous familial structures, and African slave influences. This was further reasserted during colonial rule, albeit in a different form, where Christian, especially Catholic values, played an important function in determining between men's and women's roles in society, and consequently engendering masculine dominance (Sternberg 2000; González 1996).

Indeed, it is important to consider how what Serrano Lorenzo (2012, 11) described as "the Indigenous, the African, and the Spanish" coincided in terms of developing and propelling a rejection of sexual diversity through *machismo*. Although little research has been carried out on the topic, the indigenous communities in Cuba maintained a patriarchal and polygamous value system, in which homosexuality was considered an illness that caused men to act in what was understood as a feminine manner. These indigenous systems preceded the African slave communities and value systems, which similarly viewed homosexuality as being essentially wrong, and indeed as an illness (Leiner 1994, 22; Serrano Lorenzo 2012, 13). The Spanish also contributed to this interpretation of sexual diversity, incorporating Catholic values, such as their understanding of gender roles. *Machismo* in Cuba developed as a result of this complex colonization process, and the melding of these value systems. *Machismo* was promoted within a patriarchal framework and held a clear view of what true "manliness" meant in Cuba (Formental Hernández et al. 2014).

Machismo thus refers to the idealized man as hyper-masculine, virile, strong, paternalistic, aggressive, sexually dominant, and unfaithful. The term also incorporates an understanding of women and their roles, glorifying virginity and faithfulness in wives, ignoring female sexuality, and rejecting sexual diversity (Maynard 2002; Peña 1991; Hernández 2008). As a result of this *machismo*, Cuban culture condemned homosexuality, promoted patriarchal values and largely ignored women's sexuality.

Evidence of this rejection of sexual diversity was present throughout the eighteenth and nineteenth centuries. From the early eighteenth century, when the first newspapers were published on the island, for example, homosexuality was stigmatized in the press. By the nineteenth century, homosexuality was commonly used in the press as the butt of satire, with specific vocabulary indicating non-heterosexuals, and invariably presenting homosexual behavior as weak, wrong, and effeminate (González Pagés 2010, 69–70).

One of the earliest known examples of this discrimination that was present in the press was an article titled "The Gays" ("Los maricones"), published on 9 September 1888, on the first page of the newspaper *La Cebolla* (Fowler 1998, 3). It stated that:

> Any foreigner walking through and around the streets of San Miguel in Havana would end up stunned at the sight of some incredible people: from the waist upwards they're women: but from the waist downwards, they're men. Although, from head to toe, they're neither men nor women.

The article continued,

> Should the gays of San Miguel and other streets, and the bordellos, be tolerated by the authorities? The Spartans didn't allow their deformed children to live: their essentially warrior and masculine organization rejected these useless creatures. Can the law not correct what nature messed up when creating? (Sierra Madero 2003, 12–14)

An extension of *machismo* was the role that women held in society. While men were measured by their masculinity, women were also socially obligated to fulfill their own specific gender roles—as the opposite of men. Women's sexuality was largely ignored, and there is some evidence of prejudice against women who did not fit into these socially prescribed gender roles, particularly regarding sexual diversity. While public cases regarding women were extremely rare, one example was that of Doña Enriqueta Fávez, who was put on trial for impersonating a man, Enrique Fávez. The court documents are dated 17 February 1822, and the case entitled "Criminal proceedings against Mrs Enriqueta Fávez for disguising herself as a man by wearing a suit in order to trick Mrs Juana de León whom she legally married" (González Pagés 2010, 70–71). The court documents explain that Doña Enriqueta Fávez, a Swiss woman living in Baracoa, impersonated a man and carried out a lesbian relationship with Doña Juana de León.

It is significant that the court documents refer to the lesbian relationship as "unnatural," and refer to Enriqueta Fávez as a "creature" (González Pagés 2010, 70–71). Moreover, the documents note that their actions were directly opposed to those outlined by the Church. This reference is important because it is one of the few documented cases (and perhaps the only one) of women's sexuality being discussed in such a public forum as a court. It is probable that the main reason that this case went to court was because it was challenging the widespread, popular understanding of masculinity, something that was not only considered uncomfortable but also was entirely unacceptable in nineteenth century

Cuba. This case also highlights the importance of Catholic values at the time, and the significance of gender roles of men and women within Cuban society.

Although there were some cases of prejudice against homosexual women, prejudice occurred significantly more against homosexual men, as they were more visible. Women's sexuality continued to be repressed and disregarded, and lesbianism was either ignored, or believed to be "correctable" (Smith and Padula 1996, 170). Yet, while they were often ignored within society, it is impossible to determine the precise levels of prejudice suffered by lesbians or sexually diverse women, as the subject has not been documented as extensively as it has been for homosexual men, and research on the topic is limited at best.

Another considerable aspect that shaped attitudes toward homosexuals in Cuba, although often overlooked, was the role of the United States. Particularly in the 1950s, drugs, gambling, and prostitution were commonplace in Havana and largely controlled by the Cuban élite and the United States-based organized crime syndicates (Turner 1989, 65). Preferential hiring treatment was given to homosexuals in the tourist sector, as homosexual prostitution was common, and mainly used to satisfy United States military personnel and tourists (Bowry 1989, 6). As a result, homosexuality would thus later be understood in revolutionary Cuba as an example of capitalist decadence, promoted by the United States and the élite.

The visibility of homosexual prostitutes would also work against them. It was this obvious association with capitalism and moral corruption that painted an even worse image of homosexuals in the minds of much of the Cuban populace. Although there were many other "macho" homosexuals on the island, the image focused on was that of the effeminate, decadent, weak, and morally corrupt homosexual male.

In order to understand homosexuality in Cuba, both leading up to the Revolution, and throughout revolutionary times, it is also important to consider what is meant by the term "homosexual." Traditionally the perception was that sex required both a passive (or "female") and an active role to be undertaken by the participants (Smith and Padula 1996, 170). Having sexual relations with a man was not enough for a person to be characterized as a homosexual; rather one was identified as such only if he adopted the passive or "female" role. The overarching understanding of what was "homosexual" related strictly to the passive partner (providing he was effeminate), while the other participating male's image could remain masculine and heterosexual in the eyes of others (Lumsden 1996, 32). Other perceived indications of homosexuality were effeminate mannerisms and a non-muscular physique. The idea of masculinity within the island thus played an important role in distinguishing who would be considered homosexual or truly "macho." A man could regularly have sexual relations with other men, but would not necessarily suffer from any prejudice if he were the active partner and were stereotypically macho (aggressive, athletic, and strong) (Smith 1992, 177). The active man could even reinforce his masculinity through dominating other men (Epps 1995, 232). Certainly, it was believed that macho men could not be classified as homosexual.

SEXUAL DIVERSITY IN REVOLUTIONARY CUBA

From the beginning of the Revolution, a particular appreciation of the nature of homophobia developed throughout the leadership and general population. In particular, the decades of the 1960s and 1970s proved to be charged with homophobic tendencies across the island. While the revolutionary government boasted that liberation had been achieved for all, homosexual men soon became the political "other," as depicted by Anderson (1983), as they did not fit into the nationalist ideal of being a true revolutionary. This view of creating and maintaining the "other" is further supported by Fidel Castro's June 1961 "Words to the Intellectuals" speech, in which he famously noted, "Within the Revolution everything goes; against the Revolution, nothing" (Castro 1961). In other words, the boundaries of what was considered to be within the Revolution's framework was made clear, as well as what was considered to be outside—or the "other." The government and general population sought to cleanse the country of everything believed to be outside of the Revolutionary framework, including that which was viewed as decadent and morally corrupt—a category that included homosexuals. Indeed, from the beginning, homosexuality was vehemently rejected by the Revolution.

The Penal Code, for example, maintained evident anti-homosexuality legislation throughout the 1960s and 1970s and continued to recycle laws that dated back to the Cuban Social Defense Code of 1938. In particular, it contained Article 490, which gave a prison sentence of up to six months to anyone who "habitually engaged in homosexual acts," sexually propositioned someone, or created a "public scandal" or "display" by flaunting their homosexuality (Roque Guerra 2011, 219).

The early 1960s also added new dimensions to the traditional homophobia practiced in Cuba. A major factor was that orthodoxy in western science at the time affirmed that homosexuality was a mental illness, and emphasized "curing" as an option (Turner 1989, 67). This created further issues and fear, as homosexuality was viewed in many ways as a threat against national health. The early 1960s also bred an atmosphere of mistrust and chaos in Cuba, as society became polarized. In effect, this added new layers of complication to the already multifaceted and profoundly rooted homophobia, as they were largely viewed as being among the counterrevolutionaries.

One of the main contributing factors to this climate of concern was the United States' relationship with Cuba. The 1961 Bay of Pigs invasion (referred to in Cuba as the invasion of Playa Girón), and attacks by the CIA-supported groups, resulted in a mistrustful and suspicious government, as well as a concerned general populace. The result was that those who seemed "different" or counterrevolutionary were further marginalized.

In addition, in the 1960s many homosexuals among the middle classes moved to the United States. This exodus was made possible as a result of the United States government's choice not to employ the Immigration and Naturalization Act of 1952 (which barred "sexually deviant" aliens from entering the country, as well as authorizing their expulsion) (Arguelles and Rich 1984, 698). While many left, others remained and were active supporters of the Revolution, some believing that what they would lose in sexual identity, they would gain in other social rights.

It is also important to note that homosexuality was particularly rejected in rural areas, where one's sexual preferences could not easily be hidden, and prejudice against perceived homosexuals (particularly men) was commonplace. For this reason, many gravitated toward more urban areas, such as the cities of Havana and Santiago de Cuba, where there was a greater possibility of sexual anonymity. In addition, *machismo* played a significant role in this rural/urban divide. Because *machismo* was more prevalent in rural areas, increasing in intensity and rigidity further away from the more urban areas, it was significantly more challenging to hide one's sexual preferences as well as maintaining the *machista* identity—particularly if that meant being married and having children. Largely as a result of a combination of the intensity of *machismo* in rural areas, as well as the increased anonymity offered in cities, many sexually diverse Cubans moved to the major cities. In fact, it was believed by many that homosexuality did not occur in rural areas.

For example, in 1969 education specialist Marvin Leiner interviewed Luis Allyón, who believed that there were no homosexuals in rural Cuba, and specifically, that there were no homosexual *campesinos*, as homosexuals were only to be found in the cities. He also posited that the numbers of homosexuals overall had decreased since the beginning of the Revolution. As Allyón explained,

> I know more than ten cases of homosexuals who entered the militia and by the end of the military experience left it behind and started to act normally. . . . Yes, it makes them change; you know why? Because it was the army of the period. It was the militia, not the army—but the army of the people. The activities of the militia took many people away from homosexuality. I know four who went on to get married and have families. (Leiner 1994, 22–23)

The rural/urban divide of homosexual presence thus offered a clear indication of the numbers of homosexuals who moved to urban areas. That is not to say that homosexuality was not present in rural areas, but rather that larger cites offered greater sexual anonymity, providing significantly more protection against discovery and prejudice.

As with the treatment of women in pre-revolutionary Cuba, specific gender roles for men and women persisted in revolutionary Cuba, as cultural norms perpetuated gender divisions. Prejudice against homosexuals was focused on men rather than women, largely because the *machista* culture had not yet incorporated a comprehensive (or even basic) understanding of women's sexuality. For this reason, lesbianism, particularly in the early years of the Revolution, was ignored or viewed as being in direct opposition to revolutionary values, as it indicated a moral weakness and a dishonorable character.

Lourdes Casal's study (1975) on sexually diverse women in literature in both pre-revolutionary Cuba and revolutionary Cuba highlights the continual relegation of women, particularly sexually diverse women, in Cuban society. Her comprehensive study of literature found only two minor references to lesbianism in the published work she examined. As Leiner (1994, 23) explains, "From the machismo point of view, lesbianism simply does not matter much. It does not seriously challenge machismo as long as women have no acceptable social choices other than marrying men." It would be several years before lesbianism would become a significant factor in Cuban society.

Homophobia continued unabated throughout the 1960s, increasing in momentum and intensity as the leadership and much of the general populace continued to view homosexuality as anathema to the Revolution. There were many arrests, as officials employed homophobia both as a means of social control, and of maintaining what were considered to be revolutionary values.

The first, and perhaps the most famous, "round-up" of homosexuals became known as the "Night of the Three Ps" (Bejel 2001, 97). The round-up of "pederasts, prostitutes, and pimps" occurred in 1961, in an effort to clean the streets and dissolve prostitution through sweeping arrests. The Night of the Three Ps was not specifically directed against homosexuals, but was an obvious indication of the direction that the revolutionary officials were heading. It is unclear if all of the "round-ups" occurred in cities, where the sexual deviant behavior was more visible and central, however we can assume that Havana, and to some degree Santiago de Cuba, were the focal areas.

One of Cuba's most famous writers, Reinaldo Arenas, wrote of his experience in Havana's El Morro prison. In his words,

> Homosexuals were confined to the two worst wards of El Morro: These wards were below ground at the lowest levels, and water seeped into

> the cells at high tide, it was a sweltering place without a bathroom. Gays were not treated like human beings, they were treated like beasts. They were the last ones to come out for meals, so we saw them walk by, and the most insignificant incident was an excuse to beat them mercilessly. The soldiers guarding us, who we called *combatientes,* were army recruits sent there as a sort of punishment; they found some release for their rage by taking it out on the homosexuals. Of course, nobody called them homosexuals; they were called fairies, faggots, queers, or at best, gays. The wards for fairies were really the last circle of hell. (Arenas 2001, 180–81)

By 1965 attitudes toward sexual diversity shifted, becoming even more rigid and anti-homosexual. The principal reasons for this shift were the increased polarization within Cuba, as well as international tensions, producing mistrust of the political "other" and of "counterrevolutionaries." The layers of political chaos and internal struggle created a perfect storm of mistrust, suspicion, and a need to define more clearly what was revolutionary and what was not.

The issue of the "other" was further compounded in the mid-1960s by the development of a clear vision of what a revolutionary Cuban ought to be—the "New Man." This concept was based on *conciencia*—a revolutionary consciousness based on moral principles. The "New Man" was seen as the ideal revolutionary—strong, morally incorruptible, socialist, and just. Moreover by this time the term "anti-social" had become commonplace, used to indicate anything considered to be "counterrevolutionary"—and often used to describe homosexuality. In addition, pre-revolutionary history was regularly used as "evidence" against the perceived evils of homosexuality. Because homosexuality was widely viewed as a capitalist illness or weakness, as well as a product of self-indulgence and decadence, homosexuals were viewed as being incompatible with the new vision of what a man should be. Homosexuals, particularly effeminate ones, were therefore considered insufficient revolutionaries and men, unable to realize the ideal of the "New Man."

Indeed, at the time, it was widely believed that one could not be both a homosexual (and thus almost by definition effeminate) and a revolutionary. Fidel Castro offered his own stark opinion on the matter, stating:

> Nothing prevents a homosexual from professing revolutionary ideology and, consequently, exhibiting a correct political position. In this case, he should not be considered politically negative. And yet we would never come to believe that a homosexual could embody the conditions and requirements of conduct that would enable us to consider him a true revolutionary, a true Communist Militant. A deviation of that nature clashes with the concept we have of what a militant Communist should be. But above all, I do not believe that anybody has a definitive answer to what causes homosexuality. I think the problem must be studied very carefully. But I will be frank and say that homo-

> sexuals should not be allowed in positions where they are able to exert influence upon young people. In the conditions under which we live, because of the problems which our country is facing, we must inculcate our youth with the spirit of discipline, of struggle, of work. In my opinion, everything that tends to promote in our youth the strongest possible spirit, activities related in some way with the defense of the country, such as sports, must be promoted. This attitude may or may not be correct, but it is our honest feeling. It may be in some cases a person is homosexual for pathological reasons. It would indeed be arbitrary if such a person were maltreated for something over which he has no control. You can only ask yourself, when assigning a person to a position of responsibility, what are the factors which might help that person do his job well, and what are those that might hinder him? (Lockwood 1967, 107)

Fidel Castro's statement illustrates the beliefs held by much of the leadership and populace regarding the place of homosexuality within the Revolution throughout the 1960s. That is, homosexuality was viewed as a sign of a weak moral character and was therefore completely incongruent with the ideal of a true revolutionary. Moreover, his statement supports the common assertion at the time that homosexuality could be spread to young people, or that young people could be somewhat "infected" by homosexuality. This, in effect, translated into homosexuality being considered an illness and significant health risk to the Revolution. In addition, it highlighted the continued emphasis on *machismo,* suggesting that athleticism and strength were required in order to be a good revolutionary.

The 1960s were also the decade in which the CDRs were established and developed as a means of monitoring their respective local communities. Particularly in the early 1960s, as the government was still forming, the CDRs were vital for maintaining local leadership within the revolutionary framework by functioning as social regulators. They were instituted at a time when U.S. aggression was particularly intense. Assassination attempts against Fidel Castro, sabotage, acts of terrorism—all sponsored by Washington, intent on destroying the Cuban Revolution—occurred with some regularity. The Cuban government thus called upon its population to be vigilant against any potentially counterrevolutionary acts, and to defend the revolutionary process. The original aim of the CDRs was to have one for every city block in order to monitor and prevent possible threats against the Revolution, including any "anti-social" or suspicious behavior. While it was not the principal aim of the CDRs, they did contribute to, and facilitate, homophobia in Cuba.

Indeed, for homosexuals, the CDRs became a considerable problem, as they held close ties with the Department of Revolutionary Orientation of the Central Committee (Comité Central) (CC) of the PCC, the Ministry of the Interior, the National Police, the FMC, as well as other ministries, governmental institutions, and mass organizations. They were important agents in ensuring social control, and maintained many vital roles for the health and safety of the general populace; yet, in the case of homosexuality, they largely functioned as informants. CDR members regularly provided police with information regarding homosexual activities or perceived "anti-social" behavior (Ocasio 2002, 80).

In addition, CDRs were responsible for authenticating or verifying information regarding a community member's "friends, visitors, family, biography, work history, present-day activities, participation in revolutionary programs, and overall moral revolutionary character" (Aguirre 1994, 546). Their approval was vital for university and job applicants, as well as young people wanting to join the Young Communists League (Unión de Jóvenes Comunistas) (UJC) (Bowry 1989, 6). In effect, this caused problems for homosexuals, in both professional and personal respects, as the government used the CDRs as an additional means of control.

The official 1965 Ministry of Public Health (Ministerio de Salud Pública) (MINSAP) report was demonstrative of the government's formal position on homosexuality. It stated that there was no known biological cause of homosexuality; therefore, it theorized, homosexuality was a learned behavior. The government, believing that homosexuality was a behavior that could be corrected or prevented, developed various strategies to eradicate it. These strategies would arguably become one of the most significant aspects of revolutionary Cuba's early position on homosexuality, as it was viewed as a national health issue, above all. By 1965, homophobia was officially institutionalized, with the opening of the UMAP camps. Relatively little is known about the camps, as no significant study has ever been undertaken to examine the necessary archival materials in Cuba. What is clear, however, is they were used as a means of re-education and re-orientation for men considered to be "anti-social," and among those required to participate were a significant number of homosexuals (Madero 2016).

Assessment of the numbers of people forced to work in the camps varied, though a common estimate is that there were some 60,000 (Lumsden 1996; Cabezas 2009). Reports vary, depending on the specific camps, but it is clear that participants were required to work very long days, for minimal pay, and in very poor conditions. Homosexual workers, especially those considered "flamboyant," often suffered more than others (Bejel 2001, 101). The camps sought to correct any anti-social behavior, and re-educate participants to fulfill the duties of a revolutionary. It was believed that, through intense physical labor, workers would learn the values of the "New Man," thus becoming more productive members of society (Gotkowitz and Richard 1984). As Yglesias (1968, 275–76) observed, following his experience in Cuba in the 1960s,

> These Military Units for Aid to Production were begun to take care of young men of military age whose incorporation into the Army for military training was considered unfeasible. Young men known to avoid work and study were candidates; so were known counterrevolutionaries; and also immoralists, a category that included homosexuals. How the recruitment worked was difficult to define: some were unexpectedly picked up and shipped to a camp, others were notified to report, and others were called in and warned and given a chance to defend themselves. Who denounced them? The secret police, their colleagues at their study or work center, and mainly the local Committees for the Defense of the Revolution.
>
> It should have been predictable that the recruits would not, in practice, be limited to young men of military age, that the categories of qualification would be blurred, and that their internment would not be educational but brutally punitive. This was all I knew about the UMAP; I did not make a study of it—I was loath to.

Homosexual participants were reportedly often segregated and required to work longer hours, and in poorer conditions. In a 1984 interview between Leiner and Juan Escalona, Cuban Minister of Justice, Escalona explained that camps were set up solely for gays in order to separate the "girls" from the "boys" (Leiner 1994, 29). This statement further supports evidence of attitudes toward homosexuality at the time, that considered homosexuals as lesser men, or alternatively as women, suggesting that their character required correcting.

The UMAPs ceased to be used as "re-education" camps in 1968, following significant national and international political criticism (Madero 2016). Of particular note, in 1966, several important artists and writers were going to be sent to the camps due to their perceived homosexuality. However the Writers and Artists Union (Unión de Escritores y Artistas de Cuba) (UNEAC) held an emergency meeting to defend and support their colleagues, demanding that they not be sent and subjected to such humiliating treatment. The meeting was successful, as authorities cancelled the request and the writers in question were not required to be "re-educated" (Rodríguez Boti 2003, 93). Around the same time the English novelist Graham Greene also wrote about the UMAPs. He condemned them as being immoral, and applauded the efforts made by UNEAC. He reportedly noted, "The Revolution can survive any political or economic error but not a moral one, and the UMAP was a moral error that must be corrected" (Yglesias 1968, 275). Among the other international figures that condemned Cuba's treatment of homosexuals were the American poet Allen Ginsburg and the French philosopher Jean-Paul Sartre, who compared Cuba's treatment of homosexuals to Nazi Germany's treatment of Jews (Krause-Fuchs 2007, 131; Ocasio 2002, 81).

In addition to the UMAPs, anti-homosexual attitudes were also institutionalized for children. Following the 1965 MINSAP report, which concluded that homosexuality was a learned behavior, research began on how to correct it. As noted in the report, "research as well as prevention must start very early in order to influence the mechanisms of this learning process" (Leiner 1994, 33). Research projects, as well as special educational programs for effeminate boys, were subsequently carried out to cure this perceived public health issue.

One of the primary studies on the development of homosexuality in boys was conducted in 1965 by J. Pérez Villar and his colleagues from the General Calixto García Hospital's Child Psychiatric Services, in Havana. The research group became interested in the topic after significant numbers of effeminate boys were brought to the clinic for treatment. As very little data existed in Cuban psychiatric literature or practice, they set out to research the determining factors of the development of homosexuality, and in particular effeminate behavior in boys. They studied fifty cases of those who were considered effeminate boys and fifty cases of those who were considered normal ones. The research concluded that effeminate behavior usually begins in children around age two or three, and develops as a result of insufficient immersion and participation in the socially prescribed gender roles, and in particular the lack of a father figure. The study affirmed the commonly held contention that homosexuality was learned by boys who had insufficient exposure to "real men," and who also received too much attention from their mothers. This study was important, as it provided the psychological data that homosexuality could be both prevented and cured. For many young boys, this meant that they were required to attend a special education facility in which they would learn to be men—the Yellow Brigades.

Children who were having difficulty at school were divided into groups or "brigades" for a given behavioral problem. These included those who were hyperactive and aggressive, anxious and withdrawn, wet the bed, had eating disorders or problems, or were effeminate in their behavior. Each brigade was assigned a color, with the effeminate boys being the Yellow Brigade, which ultimately sought to masculinize the boys by, among other means, forcing them to play with pistols and swords, participate in aggressive sports, and prohibiting them from doing anything considered effeminate, as well as encouraging their fathers to take a more active role in their sons' lives (Leiner 1994, 34). These programs were ongoing throughout roughly the same period as the UMAPs.

The importance of the Yellow Brigades goes beyond their being an example of institutionalized homophobia at the time, as it highlights the state's understanding of and belief in the importance of the safety and health of the general population. The children were taken out of school and placed in the brigades to cure or prevent homosexuality, in addition to preventing the spread of homosexuality to other students. This should be understood as both the government's effort to correct a perceived problem as well as an attempt to protect the rest of the population and to minimize those who were "infected." Indeed, effeminate boys, who would later grow into homosexual men and continue to infect others, were interpreted as a public health concern, illustrating the dominant belief in the importance of health and preventive healthcare in revolutionary Cuba as a means of protecting the population.

The start of the relaxation of policies regarding sexual diversity, as well as an improvement in the quality of life for homosexuals, was marked by various major events spanning the late 1960s and the 1970s. The first was East Germany's legalization of homosexual acts between adults in 1968. The Cuban government's desire to compete with what were believed to be other progressive countries drove the government to begin to reassess policies and attitudes (Arguelles and Rich 1984, 692). This was furthered by the evolution in the use of official vocabulary used for homosexuality by other countries across Western Europe and North America (Turner 1989, 70–71).

Yet, despite the Cuban government's desire to learn from the experiences of East Germany and other nations perceived as being progressive, the island's severe homophobia continued throughout the late 1960s and 1970s. Although the use of the UMAPs was phased out, anti-homosexual attitudes were institutionalized in other ways, in particular by prohibiting homosexuals from working in any field involving children in order to decrease the risk of "infection," and minimizing the visibility of homosexual or effeminate behavior. The Penal Code also continued for some time to maintain notably homophobic legislation.

An example of attitudes held at the time is an article titled "Homosexuality" ("Homosexualismo"), published on 21 February 1969 in the popular *Bohemia* magazine. Written by the Deputy Minister of Education, Abel Prieto Morales, the article explained in detail why homosexuality had to be considered a psychological illness and neurological problem. The caption below the title stated clearly the intention of the article,

> This is an essay.—Glands lose their prestige as a major causal factor.—So this is not homosexuality?—That which seems to conceptualize the basic phenomenon.—Be careful! It starts early.—Family and environment.—Difficult to reverse.—The important thing is to avoid producing the homosexual.—Do you "understand" the problem? (Prieto Morales 1969, 108)

The article was introduced with an experience the author had. The first paragraph read:

> A few weeks ago, a young, demobilized man following his obligatory military service came to our offices to complain that he had been rejected by the Regional Commission of Investigations as a potential secondary school teacher. I asked him:—Did they explain the reason?—It seems there was a problem with my past.—What kind of problem? He

> looked down and responded—A moral problem. I tried to look him in the eyes and I asked him without beating around the bush—A homosexual experience? He didn't say anything. His silence was itself an answer.

The author continued to argue that homosexuality was perverse and an illness. Citing French writer Marcel Eck's essay "Sodom. Essay on Homosexuality" ("Sodome. Essai sur l'homosexualité"), Prieto Morales argued that homosexuality should be understood as a "neurotic state," since a homosexual mind was one that had reverted back to an infantile state. The article continued to contradict authors who had argued that homosexuality was normal, using Villar's study on homosexual or effeminate boys as evidence to suggest that it was an abnormality starting when children were very young. Prieto Morales offered further evidence for his contention by explaining that homosexuality was very rare in rural areas because of all the daily activities and time spent outside. Moreover, he explained that once one engaged in homosexual behavior it was very difficult to reverse or cure (Prieto Morales 1969, 108).

As very little was published on the topic at the time, this article is important as it offered an incontrovertible example of the societal homophobia of the 1960s and early 1970s, particularly as held in government circles. The understanding was rather simplistic, and was based upon several fundamental concepts. In terms of homosexuality, women were ignored; the "condition" was believed to be more common in urban regions; and, importantly, it was seen as a preventable illness caused by a lack of macho presence in a young boy's life.

Much like the 1960s, the 1970s were characterized by repression of homosexuals. The 1971 Declaration of the First National Congress on Education and Culture significantly complicated issues regarding homosexuality, developing institutionalized homophobia, while promoting a narrowly focused form of sexual education. In essence the complication was two-fold: it promoted the need for comprehensive sexual education, while it simultaneously banned homosexuals from participating in the education process, denouncing homosexuality as a form of deviant behavior.

The Congress was held in Havana, with 1,800 delegates from across the country. It was the product of some 116,000 educational workers participating in 2,599 sessions at the municipal, regional, and provincial levels to debate the main areas regarding education (such as the role of parents and teachers, methodology, and content) (Leiner 1994, 35; UNESCO 1971, 5–6). The results were significant. The Congress recognized the importance of external influences of education, and thus promoted an increase in control over publishing on the island. The Congress also set out various parameters to ensure the exclusion of homosexuals from any positions of teaching, attempting to minimize their visibility and cultural influence, particularly on young people. Indeed the Congress adopted a resolution that considered homosexuality as "an antisocial pathology, against socialist morality" (Roque Guerra 2011, 221). Various writers and intellectuals considered to be living outside these moral parameters were required to change jobs in order to reduce their effect on the public (Rodríguez Boti 2003, 93).

These suggestions made by the Congress were officially legalized in 1974, with a law prohibiting homosexuals from working in any position in which they could influence children or young people. The new law, Law 1267, published in the *Gaceta Oficial* on 12 May 1974, was an extension of Law 1166, established on 23 September 1964. It outlined clearly the restrictions on homosexuals, as well as others engaging in socially inappropriate behavior, as they were unable to work in any position related to education, and particularly any positions that could affect or infect children or young people (Rodríguez Boti 2003, 93–94). This official ban would continue until the introduction of the 1978 Labor Law, though it would continue unofficially for some time, as it was still ingrained in many ways throughout society (Leiner 1994, 36).

The first half of the 1970s was the *Quinquenio Gris*, which was largely an extension of the restrictive policies present at the First National Congress. The period is officially seen as lasting five years, although in effect it continued for over a decade. Defensive attitudes reminiscent of those of the early 1960s returned, with the leadership concerned with ensuring the survival of the Revolution. Any manifestation of perceived opposition to the government, anything seen as being different from the narrowly focused revolutionary ethos, was considered unacceptable. Specifically, this is generally understood as a culturally repressive period, as the restrictions focused primarily on the work of some intellectuals and writers. The aim was not explicitly to bar homosexuals from cultural events and publishing, but in effect it did so in many ways, and ultimately reemphasized the country's anti-homosexual tendencies, and social regulation.

These cultural bans were established by the Congress and were present throughout the *Quinquenio Gris* until they began to be lifted in 1976 with the establishment of the Ministry of Culture (Ministerio de Cultura) (MINCULT). Following several tense years of cultural repression, MINCULT was established to engage cultural areas within the Revolutionary framework. Of particular importance, the Ministry took over the Instituto Cubano del Libro, and became a principal publisher of literature, including significant amounts on sexual education and sexual healthcare.

In terms of understanding the evolution of policies and rights regarding sexual diversity in Cuba, scholars have placed significant emphasis on the 1971 Declaration of the First National Congress on Education and Culture, and the cultural restrictions emphasized throughout the *Quin-*

quenio Gris; yet its importance has largely been misunderstood. In terms of homosexuality, scholarly work on the 1971 Congress has exclusively addressed the Congress's role in institutionalized homophobia, and not sexual education. It is important to consider that the Congress was of importance not because it offered another example of institutionalized homophobia, but rather because it strongly encouraged the need for comprehensive sexual education. Moreover, it noted the importance of external influences in education, including the media and family.

In effect, while it highlighted ongoing homophobia, the 1971 Congress would prove to be an important event in the development of sexual education and attitudes toward sexual diversity as it served to open a national debate on sexuality, and promoted sexual education. Despite the increased institutionalized homophobia, and although previously ignored by commentators until now, the Congress's emphasis on sexual education would actually become a significant means of developing the country's sexual diversity rights. Similarly, the *Quinquenio Gris* has often been interpreted as a culturally repressive time, especially for authors. However, importantly, this tumultuous period led to the establishment of MINCULT, which was responsible for large amounts of significant publications regarding sexuality.

The 1970s also continued to produce significant changes in attitudes toward, and understanding of, sexuality and gender constructions. The FMC, and in particular the development of Cuba's unique brand of feminism, was paramount to this. As a result of the FMC and its considerable influence, the Family Code was developed in 1974 and codified the following year. It was crucial in redefining gender roles in Cuba, as women sought to redefine themselves outside the rigid *machista* framework, as equals. Prior to the Family Code women were encouraged to participate within the Revolution, but were still responsible for all of the childrearing and household chores and were expected to be complacent, feminine, and were not believed to be as capable as men.

The Code called for several changes, including equal participation by both sexes in childcare and household responsibilities (Family Code 1979). This was the result of both Cuban feminism and the concept of *machismo* becoming increasingly challenged, as it no longer supported the revolutionary values regarding equality. The Code's implementation was therefore significant because it was illustrative of the evolving understanding of gender roles and the understanding of equality (more specifically, gender equality), and formally legitimated the importance of the role of women in the home as well as the workplace. Moreover, for the evolution of attitudes toward sexual diversity, the Code was historically important because it broadened and altered the understanding of gender roles. However, it was also problematic in this regard because it focused on the heteronormative nuclear family, implying that heterosexuality was the only option for families; in addition, this suggested that one needed to be heterosexual in order to be a good Cuban. Nonetheless, it successfully challenged ideas of gender roles, and would remain a critical step in the evolution of the country's attitudes toward sexual diversity.

The National Group for Work on Sexual Education (Grupo Nacional de Trabajo de Educación Sexual) (GNTES) was also established in 1972, headed by FMC president, Vilma Espín, and a Cuban physician, Celestino Álvarez Lajonchere. The aim was to devise and oversee a sweeping national sexual education effort, as well as research the latest information and theories regarding sexuality (Lumsden 1996, 101–2). The establishment of GNTES was instrumental in normalizing sexual diversity, as it opened a national debate on the topic and incorporated sexuality into healthcare.

The year 1979 was significant for various reasons. Chief among them were amendments to the Penal Code that officially decriminalized homosexuality. However, despite the official decriminalization of homosexual acts between adults, the new legislation indicated the government's continuing struggle to accept homosexuality, as it was in many ways only superficially more liberal. For example, the 1979 Penal Code contained the highly subjective and vague Law of Dangerousness (*Ley de Peligrosidad*), which sought to protect the Revolution by legally permitting the arrest of anyone considered to be counterrevolutionary. Under this section, anyone thought to be participating in any "anti-social" or "dangerous" behavior could receive sentences varying from one to four years of therapy, prison time, or payment of large fines. Moreover, until it was revised in 1987, the 1979 Penal Code prohibited "public ostentation" of a homosexual "condition" (Lumsden 1996, 82). This left many in the hands of prejudiced police and judiciaries. Thus, while homosexuality was officially decriminalized, it was still not legalized and much of the legislation remained implicitly anti-homosexual and repressive. In other words, one could legally have a homosexual relationship in private, but the legislation did not allow these relationships to be visible in public, and maintained strict regulations regarding employment opportunities of homosexuals.

In addition, the 1979 legislation that related to sex with minors was also notably homophobic. The section that dealt with "crimes against the Normal Development of Sexual Relations" outlined this clearly. Article 310 stated that an adult who provoked homosexuality in a minor male (below the age of sixteen), could receive a prison sentence of up to five years. For women, the age of consent for sexual relations was twelve; however, if they were engaging in a homosexual act, their age of consent increased to sixteen (Arguelles and Rich 1984, 693). While homosexual acts between consenting adults (in private) were officially decriminalized in 1979, the legalization of sexual diversity was a considerably more complex process.

Finally, 1979 also proved to be an important year for the gradual acceptance of, and respect for, transsexual and transgender citizens. Following various requests from the FMC, MINSAP authorized the establishment of a specialized multidisciplinary team, led by GNTES, which would provide comprehensive assistance to transgender citizens (Castro Espín 2008a; Castro Espín 2008b). As Castro Espín (2011, 27) explained, "A GNTES multidisciplinary group was set up, comprising specialists in care of transsexual persons, and the group adopted internationally approved diagnostic and therapeutic procedures, which were incorporated as services offered free of charge by the NPHS, along with courses to train sex therapists."

The aid from the multidisciplinary group originally came in health-related support, such as therapy, provision of hormones, and diagnostic procedures. As research and understanding of the topic developed, the program soon evolved into an integral treatment model that included psychological support and social integration assistance. Various ministries were involved in the newly integrated model, including MINSAP, the Ministry of Justice (MINJUS), and the Ministry of the Interior (MININT) (Acosta 2006; LeBreton 1997).

In terms of the development of surgical treatment for transgender people, the first gender-reassignment (male to female) surgery was undertaken in 1988. Although the surgery was successful, shortly afterwards it was determined that the national healthcare system did not have sufficient training in the field, or the necessary equipment to continue carrying out the surgeries. It would be twenty years before further operations were undertaken (Castro Espín 2008a; Castro Espín 2008b).

An additional important factor in the normalization of transgender citizens, albeit perhaps unintentionally instituted, was the 1985 law that allowed citizens to legally change their names. Article 43 of Law 51 of the State's Civil Registry, which was passed on 15 July 1985, allowed a citizen to change their first and last names (Fernández Martínez and González Ferrer 2008, 176). While this law was not established directly with transgender people in mind, it would serve as an important step for those participating in a non-heteronormative lifestyle to legally be who they chose to be, if only in name. Yet there is also a greater significance to changing one's name in revolutionary Cuba, as citizens are required to carry a national identification card. Although one could legally change one's name, problems would inevitably follow if the name did not necessarily match the indicated gender when required to show identification. This would cause issues with the police, physicians, and job opportunities. Nonetheless, it remains an important step in the overall normalization of sexual diversity—despite probably being an unintentional shift by the government.

The 1980 Mariel boatlift also presented a new and interesting dimension to homosexuality in Cuba. After Fidel Castro announced that those wishing to leave were allowed to do so, some 125,000 Cubans left for the United States (Epps 1995, 266). The Cuban government instituted a system whereby they were able to prioritize those who, in the eyes of the revolutionary government, were "undesirable." Among the undesirables were a number of homosexuals (alongside others, including criminals) (Peña 2007, 485). Reinaldo Arenas, who had written extensively about the abuses he received due to his homosexuality, was among those to leave (Maynard 2002).

This posed a problem for those who did not fit into one of the Government's "undesirable" categories, yet wished to leave. A common solution was then to pretend to be homosexual—particularly a "passive" homosexual. Throughout the interview process, many Cubans dressed in stereotypically homosexual and effeminate clothing (tight-fitting and colorful), emphasized their "feminine" mannerisms, and openly announced their homosexuality to officials (Peña 2007, 489). Notably, throughout the exodus, there were few lesbians in comparison to the numbers of gay males. This could be attributed to various factors, though the most likely reasons are that, as they were less visible and perhaps suffered less discrimination, they were able to integrate more easily into society, and thus did not hold the same desire to leave, or alternatively left without being categorized specifically as lesbian. Throughout the 1980s, attitudes toward sexual diversity continued to develop slowly and (at times reluctantly) to be liberalized, as the government subtly shifted its policies to become more tolerant, or at least demonstrably less discriminatory. However, while policies were less overtly discriminatory, they were rather ambiguous. By the late 1980s, policies no longer explicitly referred to homosexuality, though they adopted an unclear and somewhat muddied stance. Attitudes were clearly changing from the institutionalized homophobia and prejudice that had existed in the 1960s, but challenges undoubtedly remained.

One MINED study, which sought to better understand the views regarding sexual education and sexuality, is revealing of attitudes toward sexual diversity in the early 1980s. The final report of this study, published in 1981, included data compiled from questionnaires completed by several hundred students (between the ages of fifteen and twenty-five), parents, and teachers from across the provinces of Pinar del Rio, Matanzas, and Havana. Of the students polled, only 12 percent believed, "homosexuality should be socially accepted." Yet, curiously, 66 percent believed that "homosexuals should be punished severely and excluded from all types of social activities," while 66.7 percent also believed that "homosexuals should be allowed to participate in social activities as long as they do not negatively influence the development of children and young people" (MINED 1981). The report noted the significance of these two contradictory statistics, and suggested that a clear understanding of homosexuality still did not exist. This is certainly indicative of the ongoing national struggle regarding the acceptance of sexual diversity and the complex national debate surrounding the topic.

With regard to public opinion, one indication of change can be seen in reports in *Juventud Rebelde* that urged tolerance for homosexuality, when a decade earlier they were ridiculing it. Although, while homosexual men and women were not explicitly excluded as a result of official policy shifts, neither were they incorporated into the national identity. In other words, tolerance was urged, but sexually diverse citizens were still not incorporated into the understanding of what a good revolutionary should be; tolerance was thus advocated over respect and inclusion into the Cuban identity. For example, despite some official shifts in policies, the effeminate, ostentatious, passive homosexual man was still viewed as the "other."

Research on homosexuality also began to shift. Rather than continuing to support the contentions produced by studies in the 1960s that had suggested that homosexuality was a mental illness, new work began to be carried out. In 1986, for example, as a result of a request by Espín and Álvarez Lajonchere, a report on, and recommendations related to, homosexuality was produced (Roque Guerra 2011, 222). Very little is known about the specifics of this report, but it is telling that it was in fact carried out. Indeed, as a result of increasing knowledge in the field, particularly as a result of links with East Germany, sexuality studies were measurably advancing.

In the 1980s, international films also began exploring the topic of homosexuality in Cuba. For example, in 1988, a lesbian Latin American woman from Texas attended some classes at a film school in Havana, and made a short film that featured interviews with people in Havana of varying sexual orientations, ages, and backgrounds, on their feelings regarding homosexuality. The film, entitled *Not Because Fidel Says So*, aimed to explore the island's homophobia, discussing the participants' various experiences. The film was not overly critical of the government or of homophobia in Cuba in general; however, it did incorporate material in which homosexual men and women discussed experiences they had encountered in facing discrimination and oppression. The film had a showing at the Public Theatre in New York in 1989, but was not shown to the general population in Cuba. Similarly, the Hollywood film *The Kiss of the Spiderwoman*, which explored homosexuality, was not shown or distributed in Cuba (Leiner 1994, 51). This was unusual, as American films had regularly been shown and distributed across the island, suggesting that a government agency probably decided that it could not be shown.

While it is unclear who was involved in the decisions, or the specifics behind the rejection of the films, the fact that they were not shown is instructive, as it illustrates that the material was still believed to be inappropriate; homosexuality was still considered unacceptable. Despite the fact that in 1993 the film *Strawberry and Chocolate* (which dealt in detail with various issues surrounding homosexuality in Cuba) would be released, it was clear by the end of the 1980s that the government still did not consider the topic of homosexuality acceptable within the Revolution.

In Las Villas, on the fifteenth anniversary of the attack on the Moncada barracks in 1968, Fidel Castro stated that, "To live in a communist society is to live without selfishness, to live among the people, as if every one of our fellow citizens were really our dearest brother" (Leiner 1994, 26). Yet in revolutionary Cuba from 1959 to 1989, it was clear that homosexuals were not amongst those who were to be treated as a "brother."

Homosexuality would be officially taken off the World Health Organization's (WHO) list of mental illness on 17 May 1990. It was an event that would affect attitudes toward sexual diversity around the world—particularly in Cuba. Leading up to this change in Cuba, however, a significant driving force would prove to be the Federation of Cuban Women (FMC). The organization would redefine sexual education and its role in the normalization of sexual diversity.

TWO

The FMC and the Development of Sexual Education and Sexual Health, 1959–1989

The development of the role of women in revolutionary Cuba has become known as "the Revolution within the Revolution" (Santana 2013, 12). Women undoubtedly became a force within the Revolution, directing and implementing change. The principal means through which they did so was the FMC, and among the initial changes was a dramatic increase in national debate regarding sexual and reproductive health, as well as sexuality. This included the development of the legal right to safe and free abortions, access to contraceptives, and the overall development of sexual education across the island. This remains, however, a largely untold story.

Much of the literature regarding women and the FMC in the early years of the Revolution discusses, among other issues, the role of women in the literacy campaigns, childcare facilities, and clothing-making courses (Randall 1974, 1978; Díaz Vallina 2001). Yet, what has not been explored in detail is the FMC's role in promoting sexual education and sexual health, and ultimately contributing significantly to the normalization of sexual diversity. In fact, the FMC has been essential in the complex development of these respective areas, but in terms of the sexual diversity rights, its significance largely lies with its role in the development of sexual health through education, and in particular establishing the link between discrimination and health—the foundation for the normalization of sexual diversity.

The FMC was established on 23 August 1960, when Fidel Castro sought to establish an organization in which women could be a "force" used to advance the Revolution (Espín et al. 2012a; Castro 1980). According to those present he explained in some detail what he believed the role of women in the Revolution should be, emphasizing the importance of women in social development. The organization soon evolved, increasing in numbers and influence, and by the 1980s, 80 percent of women over the age of fourteen were members, and the organization arguably enjoyed the same level of power as a Ministry. This influence was employed to promote and develop projects it believed were important to the Revolution and the well-being of the population.

It is worth noting that feminism in Cuba differs from other forms of feminism. While it has not been studied at length, it is clear from interviews and analyses of the FMC's literature that, rather than focusing on gender equality, Cuban feminism (as expressed by and through the FMC), particularly in the 1960s and 1970s, focused on equal participation in the Revolution, and its development. Moreover, terms such as "gender equality" and "feminism" were not used in official communications for the first decades of the Revolution, as the FMC and the island's feminist discourse focused instead on the full "participation" of all (PCC 1976; Espín et al. 2012b; Randall 1992, 1978; Valdés Stable 1977; Proveyer Cervantes et al. 2011).[1] Indeed Cuban feminism does not fit comfortably into the then-established framework of Marxism (Chinchilla 1991; Engels 1972; Bandarage 1984; Barrett 1980; Hartmann 1981). The same can be said about its difference with socialist, liberal, or even Third World feminism (Haraway 2000; Bhavnani and Coulson 1986; Baksh-Soodeen 1998; Wendell 1987; FMC 1998).[2] For example, the founders of the FMC did not even describe themselves as feminists, but rather as proponents of equal participation of men and women at all levels of society—in the home, sugarcane fields, university, and leadership (Aguilar Ayerra[3] 2013 [Interview]).

Feminism in Cuba developed based on revolutionary ideology, and continued to evolve as a result of the specific challenges that faced the Revolution at any given time. The FMC, as well as Cuban feminism, must thus be understood as promoting participation throughout the revolutionary process, above all (FMC 1962; 1975; 1987). Women sought to participate in the Revolution, and as a result have had a significant role in shaping it.

It is also worth considering the understanding of sexuality in Cuba. Although only marginally different from the interpretations developed by the works of Kinsey et al. (1948; 1953), Foucault (1990a; 1990b; 1990c), and Masters and Johnson (1966), among others, which largely discussed sexuality as different forms of sexual orientation, the Cuban view is more wide-ranging. The understanding of "sexuality" in Cuba refers to all aspects of sex; in other words, it includes how one engages with the physical act of sex. Much like "sexual diversity," the use of the term "sexuality" can therefore be understood as an umbrella concept that goes beyond sexual orientation, and includes all physical and emotional aspects of sex.

By incorporating sexuality into the national debate and establishing the link between discrimination against women's sexuality and health rates, the FMC was able to create significant change in the fields of sexual education and sexual health. This, ultimately, would lay the groundwork for further advancements in the normalization of sexual diversity.

THE FMC'S FIRST NATIONAL CONGRESS: EMPHASIZING EDUCATION

When examining the evolution of sexual education and sexual health in Cuba from the 1960s, it is instructive to note the role of the FMC, and in particular its early commitment to sexual education. Before the Revolution, sexual education was not a priority of the government, and was absent from the formal education system. Curricula in schools incorporated, depending on the age of students, aspects of the female and male anatomy and reproductive systems, but omitted the concepts of family planning and sexuality (Maderos Machado 1994).

The FMC was therefore of paramount importance in the establishment and development of reproductive and sexual health. It had become clear within the government that there was a significant lack of medical and educational attention paid to reproductive and sexual health. The FMC incorporated these topics into its development, attaching significant national importance to the improvement of sexual health. In essence, in the 1960s, many women participating in the FMC decided for themselves that better sexual health was needed, and worked through the FMC to achieve this (FMC 1962). In FMC meetings at the various levels, for example, women noted the need for sexual education. As they had little understanding themselves, they wanted to know how to educate their children on the topic (Aguilar Ayerra 2013 [Interview]).

The FMC's 1st National Congress, held in 1962, was important because it highlighted three of the organization's main responsibilities, and those of Cuban women in general. These were: improving the country's public health system and healthcare; continuing to develop education across the island; and promoting the participation of women in the revolutionary process. It was clear from the Congress that healthcare and education were among the priorities for Cuban women, and by extension their families. As the opening address noted, "As our program states, it is necessary to forge a new woman, one born out of a socialist society who enjoys all the resulting rights, actively incorporated into the workforce, freed from domestic slavery and the weight of prejudices from the past" (FMC 1962, 10).

The development and maintenance of public health in particular was a principal topic at the 1st Congress. For example, within the Commission of Social Services (Comisión de Servicios Sociales), there was a section titled "Public Health," which noted,

> It is a task of enormous importance to protect the health of our people, and in order to meet this goal the active participation of the masses is necessary—bringing the essential elements to the population in order to protect the population's health and prevent disease. (FMC 1962, 36–37)

Discussions at the Congress also highlighted a unique understanding of "education." Rather than providing a focus on the school curricula, the concept of education was presented as the means through which information was communicated to and absorbed by all; i.e. education should be seen as a broad concept that refers to the process through which information is distributed and interpreted within the revolutionary structure. This included, for example, what was referred to as "revolutionary education" ("instrucción revolucionaria"), which meant the continued communication of revolutionary values, such as the importance of equality (FMC 1962, 47).

In terms of sexual education and healthcare, the most important discussion at the Congress was about the development of a comprehensive sexual education program. The FMC suggested a need to incorporate sexual education within various areas, including the media, research, and publications, as well as in the school system. This was such a strongly held position that Fidel Castro requested that the Minister of Education attend the discussion (Aguilar Ayerra 2013 [Interview]).

EARLY RESULTS OF FMC EFFORTS: *MUJERES*, ABORTION, AND CONTRACEPTION

The origins of the normalization of sexual diversity can be found in the FMC and its work in the areas of sexual education and sexual health. Through a focus on developing abortion rights, making relevant information available, and developing contraception, the FMC enabled sexuality to become central to the national debate on health. This undoubtedly established the building blocks of the normalization of sexual diversity in later years.

Among the concerns put to the FMC in the early years of the Revolution was the lack of sexual education, particularly pertaining to reproductive health and contraception. While the FMC had paid significant attention to some areas such as the distribution of contraception beginning in 1960, there was a general feeling that this approach was insufficient. Women had noted in meetings at all levels that this was a significant problem, requesting that the FMC work toward improving the scarce resources. Similar concerns were brought up about abortion rights, as in the vast majority of cases it was illegal to terminate a pregnancy, until 1965 when it was legalized as a result of FMC efforts. Moreover, due to abortions being largely illegal, as well as a lack of trained specialists available, self-administered abortions were common—making it a noticeable health issue. The 1st Congress confirmed the national need for a dramatic increase in sexual and reproductive education, as well as the need for safe and legal abortions.

One of the most influential means by which the FMC distributed information and engaged with women across the country was a bi-monthly magazine focusing on women—*Mujeres*. The first edition of the magazine was published on 15 November 1961. *Mujeres* would become a vital channel of communication throughout the island, as the FMC employed it to convey information, which gradually increased in the area of sexual and reproductive education. As Aguilar Ayerra noted, "before the Revolution women had had little opportunity to learn about healthcare, nutrition, clothing choices, or socialist ideology, but the widespread distribution of *Mujeres* effectively changed that" (Aguilar Ayerra 2013 [Interview]).

The magazine was published by the FMC, after the women's magazine aimed at middle-class women (*Vanidades*) changed ownership and started to be run by the revolutionaries. It was the most important of the magazines directed toward women (another popular magazine was *Romances*, which later became *Muchachas*). Particularly during the early years of the Revolution, the magazine was a vital means of distributing information to women and was especially important in the rural areas (Aguilar Ayerra 2013 [Interview]).

The roots of the new direction of the magazine can be found in the FMC's 1st National Congress, when it was agreed that such a magazine was needed. As outlined at the Congress, "We do not want to publish a magazine filled with dogma, but rather one that guides women. Nor do we want a magazine filled with ideas that are incomprehensible for the majority of women—but rather we want one that is readable, instructive, and educational in all of its sections" (FMC 1962, 21). The influence of the magazine continued to increase, as it developed into an educational fixture of the FMC. Discussions regarding its contents were an invariable aspect of all FMC Congresses, and the content was continually adapted to fit what the perceived needs of women were.

In terms of normalizing sexual diversity, the most important aspect of the magazine was its role in providing basic sexual education and information regarding sexual health, which translated into increased discussion of sexuality within the national debate. A section called "Debates on Health" (*Debates de salud*) was specifically created to teach women about their own health and bodies. The magazine editors (among them founders of the FMC, including Isabel Moya and Aguilar Ayerra) contacted medical specialists to write the section in an effort to increase the depth of information, as well as emphasize the correct use of terminology of the sexual organs. The section was located at the back, typically a two-page spread with a photograph or drawing, as well as descriptions or definitions (FMC 1973a, 1973b). Importantly, the content was not written using complex wording or phrasing, allowing the information to be accessible and available to a wide audience.

The FMC's belief in the importance of *Mujeres* as an educational tool for women throughout the country is illustrated by some of the methods of distribution. As Aguilar Ayerra explained, "I remember we had to send planes to drop off packets of the magazines in the Sierra. We did that all over the mountains. It was important that all women read the magazine, not just the ones in urban parts of the country" (Aguilar Ayerra 2013 [Interview]). The exact number of the magazines distributed across the island is unknown, however we do know that the FMC went to great lengths to ensure that as many women as possible had access to the information.

The FMC's success in legalizing abortions was also tremendously important. Notably, the FMC developed abortion rights by employing a health-based approach, while also asserting that women had a right to control their own bodies, unlike in capitalist societies, which it believed commodified and controlled women.

Yet while the FMC employed an argument that centered on women's rights within the Revolution, the de-criminalization of abortions and eventual societal acceptance of abortions across the island were largely the result of placing the issue within a health framework. In other words, when it was argued that abortions could significantly reduce maternal and infant mortality, it became easier to convince the government's Ministries and the National Assembly, as well as the general populace, of the importance of safe and legal abortions. Health in this context was the defining argument used to change decades-old beliefs toward abortion rights.

The process by which abortions became legalized was complex. Under Spanish colonial rule, under the 1879 Penal Code, abortion in Cuba was illegal. Amendments were made in 1938 to the Social Defense Code, in which Article 443 established that no criminal charges would be applied in certain circumstances:

> Abortion is necessary to save the life of a mother, or to avoid serious damage to her health; when it is carried out, with the mother's consent, as a result of the crime of rape, pregnancy of an unmarried woman as a result of forced or coerced intercourse and intercourse with a minor; when it is carried out with the consent of the parents with the aim of avoiding transmission to the fetus of a serious hereditary or contagious disease. (Álvarez Lajonchere 1994, 6–7)

At the beginning of the Revolution, attitudes toward abortion remained negative, particularly in rural areas, and the 1938 law continued to be enforced. Problems with medically safe abortions also increased in the early years of the Revolution, as half of Cuba's 6,000 physicians (many of whom were specialists, including gynecologists, obstetricians, and *aborteros* as they were commonly known) left the island.

Álvarez Lajonchere remembered the negative health effects that occurred as a result of the illegality of abortion. He explained that many women, especially those who had limited financial resources, resorted to self-induced abortions. He noted that, even growing up in a small town—la Moza, Manicaragua in Villa Clara province—he and everyone knew about the clinic in Cienfuegos that performed abortions, if the patient could afford the service and medication, despite it being illegal. He asserted that across the country, very little was understood about abortions, and it was unclear how many took place, or what the possible side effects would be. As he explained,

> Between 1960 and 1965 we witnessed some terrible things, some of which I will NEVER forget. The insertion into the uterus of clothes hangers and especially the use of intrauterine douches using a variety of ingredients are examples of this. The most popular was "cundiamor," a plant with a fleshy fruit belonging to the same family as the pumpkin, melon and cucumber. When these mixtures do not cause complications resulting in sepsis, the intrauterine douche is effective in interrupting the pregnancy. The cases where sepsis did not result were in the minority.
>
> In several cases if the women were young they would use a solution of sulphuric acid (Salfuman is the brand name, and it is used as a cleaning solution in public toilets). When I asked a young woman who appeared to be in good health, but who had undergone this treatment about this, and examined her with a vaginal speculum it was clear that very little remained of the fetus "there." Without exception, a few hours later they were dead. (Álvarez Lajonchere 1996, 28–29)

During the early years of the Revolution, many of the causes of maternal mortality were reduced, but unsafe abortions still posed some severe problems for maternal and child health (Álvarez Lajonchere 1994, 28–29). By 1965, it had become clear that the problem needed to be addressed.

Legislation was changed as a result of the significant health issues caused by unsafe abortions, as well as the exclusion of many women from the opportunity to participate in the Revolution due to caring for unplanned or unwanted children. In particular, MINSAP re-interpreted the 1938 legislation to allow all early-term abortions (Álvarez Lajonchere 1994, 6–7). Moreover, it established that abortions would be provided free of charge to patients, and in medically sound facilities. By 1979, the 1938 legislation had been completely re-written, and provided additional legal support for abortion rights, although approval had to be given by the hospital's director if a woman sought an abortion in the second or third trimesters.

Espín explained in a 1997 edition of *Mujeres* entitled, "Architects of Their Own Destiny,"

> We soon won the right to have abortions included as a service of the health system, legalized under [the] condition that they be performed by specialists and in hospitals, assuring all necessary sanitary conditions. The Federation then called on the country's health and education institutions to carry out massive educational efforts and to organize a genuine program of sexual education, open to all and based solidly on advanced scientific concepts. (Espín et al. 2012c, 235; FMC 1997, 4)

Throughout the debate and legalization process, the most significant argument used was that of the health-based approach. In particular, it was argued by the FMC that many abortions occurred in adolescents, who have significantly higher infant and maternal mortality rates, as well as general health issues related to pregnancies. Moreover, unsafe abortions are likely to create further health issues for the mother, increase infant mortality rates, as well as create further health problems in future pregnancies (Álvarez Lajonchere 1994, 6–7; Álvarez Lajonchere 1996, 25–29; Prendes Labrada 2007).

Undoubtedly, the most important contribution of this health-based approach was the establishment of the discrimination-health link. While abortions were de-criminalized, many women felt uncomfortable undergoing the procedure as a result of the societal discrimination and prejudice that they would encounter (being viewed as too sexually active, not a virgin, or irresponsible). Women continued to self-administer abortions, despite the considerable health risks, in order to avoid the discrimination that they would likely face for having the procedure done by a professional. It was believed that the discrimination facing these women was clearly linked to their health rates, and by extension national health rates. As a result, the FMC began to increase its efforts to normalize sexuality and sexual health, employing the discrimination-health link to increase the national debate of sexuality and improve sexual education and sexual health, with the ultimate aim of normalizing abortions. The considerable health issues faced by the women and children as a result of the societal prejudices associated with abortions was enough to convince the government and eventually the majority of the population that abortions should not be discriminated against. The implementation of the discrimination-health link was a strategy that clearly worked well in the Cuban context.

Data suggest that abortions in Cuba have proved to be a significant means of reducing rates of infant mortality and maternal mortality, as well as a means of family planning (Sosa Marín 1994, 10–11). For example, from 1968, when the government began compiling statistics on abortions, to 1992, approximately 2.9 million abortions were performed, while 4.7 million live births were registered (Alfonso Fraga 1994, 8–9). The number of abortions has continued to increase. A Cuban study published in 1996 noted an increase from 1970: in 1970, 70,521 abortions were carried out (36.1 abortions for every 1,000 women), but by 1975, 126,107 abortions were carried out (57.4 abortions per 1,000 women), though the rates would decrease by 1986 to 160,926 abortions (50.6 abortions per 1,000 women) (Peláez and Rodríguez 1996).

It should also be noted that the vocabulary regarding abortions changed significantly. While they were originally known as "abortions," the colloquial vocabulary shifted to refer to them as "interruptions." The shift was subtle, but the euphemism attached to "interruption" was clear. The change occurred following the legalization process, and efforts were made to decrease the stigma related to abortions; the vocabulary changed to minimize the shame and embarrassment often faced by the women undergoing the procedure, and thus the discrimination that was associated with it. Sexual education promoted by the FMC highlighted a woman's sovereignty over her own body, and thus it was argued that there was no reason to feel ashamed about wanting or having an abortion (Aguilar Ayerra 2013 [Interview]; Castro Espín 2013 [Interview]). Although abortion as a means of contraception was, and remains, strongly discouraged, rates have remained high across the island.

Another means through which the FMC normalized sexuality from the 1960s was the use and distribution of contraception. Comparatively few means of contraception were available throughout the 1960s, and they were often of poor quality; condoms, for example, were imported from China, but were badly made and uncomfortable to wear. Due to the United States' embargo, oral contraceptives were also very difficult for the government to import, and thus the use of other options was encouraged. Moreover, persisting cultural norms (such as women feeling uncomfortable touching their genitals) dissuaded many women from using the diaphragms (commonly known as *sombrillas*) that were ordered by MINSAP. IUDs were among the most popular form of birth control at the time due to having the fewest side-effects, and the FMC reportedly made their own cost-effective versions with nylon fishing line until the 1980s, when manufactured versions were imported. Yet birth control in the 1960s was still in many ways stigmatized and not fully incorporated into the healthcare system. For example it was uncommon for doctors to inquire about sexual history or suggest contraceptives. Rather, women had to specifically and directly inquire about options for birth control. This, for many women, was a highly uncomfortable conversation, especially due to the ongoing stigmatization of sexually active women. Alternatively, many women were largely unaware of birth control as an option, and would thus not inquire, due to a simple lack of knowledge (Smith and Padula 1996, 71; Randall 1981, 69).

In 1964 the FMC and MINSAP began working with, and receiving assistance from, the International Family Planning Program (Programa

Internacional de Planificación Familiar) (IPPF). Through the IPPF, Cuba was able to import much-needed contraceptives, while also developing a greater understanding of family planning, including education (Castro Espín 2013 [Interview]).

Although there were some problems surrounding the use of contraception, from the 1960s, the government did gradually make contraception and related information available across the island, and by the end of the 1970s the situation had improved significantly. Cuba was manufacturing its own birth control pills, and diaphragms were more commonly recommended by physicians and used by patients (Álvarez Lajonchere 1996, 26).

The development of contraceptives was also important for women, because it allowed them to engage more safely in a healthy sexual life, while minimizing the risk of unwanted pregnancy. The emphasis of the FMC on safe sexual practices was also an important component in this process, as it pressured the government to produce the necessary birth control and information to protect women's health. The medicalization of sex in the 1960s also supported the FMC's emphasis on the importance of sexual education and sexual health as a significant aspect of an individual's personal development.

Today these accomplishments are still lauded in Cuba and considered to be examples of the early influence of the FMC. *Mujeres* would continue to evolve, as well as its sister magazine, *Muchachas,* which focused on adolescent women. The magazine would also publish material from popular sexual education books, and later established a new section titled Let's Speak Frankly (*Hablemos francamente*), which in essence was a newer version of *Debates de salud* to reflect contemporary sexual education needs (FMC 1984b; Revalo 2002). The new section was most often written by the FMC representative and expert in sexuality, Aloyma Ravelo, and topics included STIs, the importance of a full sexual life, prejudices related to sexuality, men's sexuality, and marital problems (Ravelo 2007a; Ravelo 2007b; Ravelo 1999; De la Cuesta 1997; Egües Cantero 1997). As the title suggests, the section discussed sexuality in a very frank and open manner, highlighting it as a normal and important aspect of one's life, personal development, and overall health. For example, as Ravelo (2002)[4] explained, "There is no doubt that throughout history—from the most ancient times to future times—eroticism has been a human necessity."

THE FMC, SEXUAL EDUCATION AND SEXUAL HEALTH, 1972–1989

The FMC and the Founding of GNTES, 1972

Following the 1960s and the demand for sexual education and sexual healthcare, the FMC began a group with the specific aim of researching options for, and information regarding, the provision of sexual education. It was founded in 1972 by Espín and Álvarez Lajonchere, and named GNTES (Castro Espín 2009, 3). Espín was a major actor in this effort, since, as the president of the FMC, she understood the need for sexual education and sexual health, a topic that was consistently brought up in FMC meetings. Moreover, as a well-known figure and leader in the Revolution, she had a significant level of autonomy, and headed the nation-wide framework of the FMC through which change could be instituted (FMC 2008, 57). The group would be fully legitimated and recognized by the state in 1977, but from 1972 it functioned solely as an FMC initiative. It slowly grew in personnel and importance, as the need for sexual education became more evident, and the FMC continued to pursue the means to develop it. Sexual education was understood by GNTES as the means of improving sexual health.

Álvarez Lajonchere had been working with the FMC since the 1960s and was also passionate about the need for sexual education in Cuba. Having grown up in a small town, he understood the difficulties faced by much of the populace, including poverty and inequality regarding healthcare and education. Following the rebellion, he remained in Cuba, with a medical practice in Havana. His work, which focused primarily on health issues related to abortions, convinced him of the importance of sexual and reproductive healthcare and education. He began working with the FMC as an advisor for the *Debates de salud* section of *Mujeres*, and as a result of his early work with the FMC and his dedication to health, he became a vital member of the original FMC-led group that sought to dramatically change the landscape of Cuban sexual education and healthcare. As he explained,

> We began with just four people—the President, a Coordinator, who was our liaison with the FMC, a secretary and a driver. Later a German translator joined us. We tried to develop an intersectoral group, in which professionals from organizations working in various topics related to sexuality participated. The group had to be, and in fact was, interdisciplinary in its approach, since this is necessary in such complex matters, particularly with regards to the treatment provided in terms of education, diagnosis, and therapy. (Álvarez Lajonchere 1996, 26)

The German translator mentioned was Monika Krause. She became involved with GNTES due to the country's relationship with East Germany. She had previously worked as a translator and interpreter for the FMC, and was thus originally asked by Espín to join GNTES to assist with similar work (Castro Espín 2013 [Interview]; Krause-Fuchs 2007, 68). Whereas she was once briefly the director of the group, officially her capacity was as coordinator and she was often "the face" of the group in interviews and meetings, as well as running seminars and appearing on sexual education television programs. It is unclear why she left Cuba in 1990, but her contribution to the evolution of sexual education was considerable.

With the principal contributors in place, GNTES sought to develop a comprehensive national program, named the National Sexual Education Program (Programa Nacional de Educación Sexual) (ProNes) (Castro Espín 2013 [Interview]; Castro Espín 2011, 26). In order to accomplish this, they began researching other countries' sexual education programs and curricula with the aim of adopting them for the Cuban system. They also sought advice from international specialists in the field. By chance, and as a result of her being a native German speaker, Krause discovered from her research in the area a curricula developed by an East German specialist in sexual education, K. R. Bach. He had developed, over an eight-year period in the late 1960s and early 1970s, sexual education curricula for high schools (Krause-Fuchs 2007, 72–72). This development led to considerable interchanges between Cuba and East Germany as GNTES sought to develop an integral and multidisciplinary sexual health education program. As the two countries were very close ideologically, and had similar political systems, and in addition since East Germany was considered by Cuba to be an advanced country, GNTES began working closely with East German specialists throughout the 1970s. While one might view this as politically significant for Cuba, it should be noted that the exchanges in sexual education resulted from East German specialists, and K. R. Bach in particular, being willing to provide information in the field of sexual education, while other specialists from other countries were not.

GNTES was founded in 1972, not 1976 or 1977 as was previously believed.[5] The discrepancy is probably due to the limited research that has been carried out on the group, and in particular to limited access to archives and personnel. The difference in dates is important because it illustrates that GNTES was not a product of the substantial official changes related to gender rights, as has been previously understood, but in fact *preceded* them. These changes include the establishment of the Family Code (1975), as well as reports presented at the 1st PCC Congress (1975) such as the "Thesis: Full Incorporation of Women in Society." It illustrates that an FMC-developed group, despite being small, was formed with the aim of researching sexual education before women and men even held a legal status of equality in the home. Indeed this original group dramatically changed the landscape of sexual education and sexual health in Cuba, and would continue to do so.

The FMC and the (Re)Founding of GNTES, 1977

The emphasis on sexual education increased in the late 1970s. Notably, formal recognition of GNTES followed the FMC's 2nd Congress that had emphasized "The Role of the Family in Socialism," which outlined the importance of the family in education (FMC 1975, 61). Sexual education became a core component of this education, and was used to promote the importance of both gender equality and health.

As a result of the PCC and the FMC's emphasis on the importance of education, the National Assembly (Asamblea Nacional del Poder Popular) (Parliament) established a Commission with the principal aim of publishing works on sexual education and sexual health. It was titled, The National Assembly's Permanent Commission On the Attention to Infancy, Youth, and the Equality of Rights of Women.[6] It worked mainly through GNTES, although also collaboratively with MINSAP, MINED, and the UJC (FMC 1982, 21–22). The Commission was initially established at the 1st PCC Congress (1975), and later expanded at the 2nd Congress (1980) (PCC 1980a; 1980b).

GNTES, which was officially recognized by the state in 1977, became the representative group of the Commission, through which it published literature on sexual education and gradually incorporated other means of education. In 1981, Espín became the president of the Commission, as the FMC assumed further control of the sexual education program, and was able to work with an increased level of independence within the revolutionary framework (FMC 2008, 55). Its main goal was to continue developing ProNes. As explained at the 3rd FMC Congress in 1980,

> In reality [GNTES] is carrying out systematic work that encompasses the basic information and guidance materials, as well as the development of a framework to train specialists in the field of medicine, psychology and education, principally with an eye to the proper preparation of personnel who, in the future, will be responsible for sexual education, as well as the treatment and therapy of sexual problems. During the course of this year the first books that deal with these topics have been published.
>
> Evidently it is necessary to strongly emphasise these aspects of sexual education precisely because so little is known about this field, and why it is here that the strongest prejudices, erroneous criticisms, and obsolete conceptions, that we should eradicate, exist. (FMC 1984a, 65)

There was a clear emphasis on dispelling all prejudices relating to sexuality through education, as well as the need to discuss sexuality within a health framework. The FMC sought to continue increasing the breadth of sexual education, and to develop its aims from researching and publishing material to integrating sexual education more fully into other disciplines. Sexual education was clearly interpreted as a means of directing social change—with the aim of improving overall health, and promoting equality.

Throughout the 1980s, GNTES and the FMC, working in collaboration with MINSAP and MINED (among others), continued to produce significant amounts of research and publications on sexual education and sexual health. In addition to the literature that was produced, the group also designed and ran courses, conferences, seminars, debates, round-tables, and presentations on sexual education, sexual health, and sexuality. These were directed at various groups including parents, teachers, and students of all levels. The courses, often held in schools, community centers or FMC meetings, discussed human sexuality, including psychological and social aspects, as well as biological influences.

The consistent themes of these education processes were respect, equality, and health (FMC 1987, 20). Among the principal topics discussed were safe and respectful sexual relations, contraception, and problems (including medical and social) related to teenage pregnancies (CENESEX 2001, 33–36; FMC 1987, 20–21; PCC 1980a, 15–18). Moreover, the group specifically trained "sex education extension workers selected from among doctors, teachers, psychologists, health officials, and specialists; the FMC; the education sector; and youth organizations at national and territorial levels" (Castro Espín 2011, 26). The intention was clear: to train the people with influence within GNTES' ProNes framework, and thus propel their vision of a comprehensive sexual education.

Another important step was the introduction in 1980 of sexual education in teacher-training colleges, universities and day-care training centers. While offered only as an optional course, it did mark a significant shift, as this represented an official course offered to those who would go on to instruct others, and especially children and young people. Moreover, in the 1980s, GNTES also began working with the other state organizations and Commissions that dealt with HIV/AIDS, with information on the infection being incorporated into the sexual education strategy by the late 1980s (McPherson Sayú 1995, 7–9).

GNTES was involved in other sexual health-based groups and Commissions. In terms of developing sexual diversity rights and healthcare, in 1979, for example, following a request by the FMC, MINSAP approved the creation of a multidisciplinary team to assist with the diagnosis and care of members of the transgender community. Led by GNTES, the team was named the National Commission on Sexual Orientation and Therapy (Castro Espín 2008b, 15–43).

In 1985, GNTES was also responsible for the creation of the Cuban Multidisciplinary Society for the Study of Sexuality (Sociedad Cubana Multidisciplinaria para el Estudio de la Sexualidad) (SOCUMES). SOCUMES was composed of various specialists, with the aim of conducting further research in areas related to sexuality, as well as developing links with other international organizations and the scientific community (Roque Guerra 2011, 222). SOCUMES also became an active member of the Latin American Federation of Sexology. This development of a multidisciplinary group also demonstrates the ongoing emphasis on expanding research, and the view of sexuality being an important aspect of personal development, particularly related to one's overall health.

In 1987, at a round-table discussion between members of GNTES and representatives from *Juventud Rebelde,* Espín explained that, through the Commission, GNTES had expanded its work, and in particular strengthened its relationship with East German specialists (Krause 1988, 7–9). Cuban specialists continued to travel to East Germany, to learn about their sexual education strategies and educational material, and to analyze which of them were applicable to the Cuban context. MINCULT was also involved from the late 1970s, as it was responsible for publishing the work that was brought back by the Cuban researchers.

Notably, GNTES members, including Álvarez Lajonchere and Krause, were central to the translation of the East German works that were published in Cuba. Among the most important and popular books were the works of Siegfried Schnabl, and East German pediatrician and specialist in sexuality, Heinrich Brückner. All the books translated and published incorporated socialist ideology, focusing on equality, and were written for parents, teachers, young people, and children. These books would become paramount in sexual education and sexual healthcare across the island, as well as vital to the incorporation of sexual diversity into the national debate.

The National Assembly's use of GNTES as the actual working entity of the Commission highlights the national importance placed on sexual education and sexual health, as well as the importance of the group itself. Their research regarding improved sexual education strategies was clearly understood as necessary and important. Indeed, it is significant that many of the books that GNTES published around this time are still widely read in Cuba today.

GNTES' SEXUAL EDUCATION AND SEXUAL HEALTH LITERATURE

As previously noted, the circumstances in which GNTES was established have often been misunderstood. A significant contributing factor was there was little, if any, evidence in the 1970s and early 1980s that the group existed at all. For example, from 1972 to 1979 there was no mention of the group or its work in either the popular *Bohemia* magazine, or *Granma* daily newspaper. In addition to the lack of presence in print, as much of the group's work was accomplished through discussions, presentations, and meetings, there are little extant data on the group. This translates into little evidence of the initial changes that occurred as a result of its efforts, or the specific information that it sought to communicate. Yet beginning in the early 1980s, subtle indications of the group's work began to emerge, such as in *Mujeres*, where, in addition to articles that focused on sexual and reproductive health, large excerpts of what were referred to as "popular-science" books (which presented scientific information in a accessible format and were widely read) that the group had published can be found. It was through the publication of popular-science books that GNTES communicated much of its work throughout the island. These publications prompted national debate, and dramatically changed sexual education and sexual health in Cuba.

The authors of these works were invariably East German, as well as noted trained sexologists or medical professionals, and among the most published were the works of Schnabl and Brückner. They wrote popular-science books that sought to increase the discussion of the concept of sexuality, as well as contribute to sexual education and sexual health. These publications were of particular importance because they presented sexuality as normal human behavior, dispelling related prejudices. The aim was to educate the reader by increasing the understanding of sexuality, while emphasizing respect and equality in a socialist framework, particularly by emphasizing the importance of health and well-being.

The first book published was Schnabl's *Man and Woman in Intimacy* (*El hombre y la mujer en la intimidad*). The book was originally published in East Germany in 1978, and published in Spanish in Cuba in 1979. It was reprinted in Cuba in 1985, and a second edition was later published in 1989 (Schnabl 1989). The publishing process in Cuba was significant, as the technical revision was done by GNTES leaders Álvarez Lajonchere and Krause, and published by MINCULT, rather than MINED or MINSAP. CENESEX Director, Castro Espín, explained that her mother and GNTES founder, Espín, had reported that at times there had been some resistance to the group publishing some works, and noted that Espín had been obliged to try various approaches in order to get the work published. Notably, it was the PCC that allocated the task of publishing GNTES' work to MINCULT (Castro Espín 2013 [Interview]). Although perhaps working with other ministries or committees, unlike the books that were published in later years, *Man and Woman in Intimacy* made no mention of other participants in the publishing process. As it was one of the first books on sexual education, and the first to discuss homosexuality in a respectful and empathetic way, which led to significant reactions from the population, it is possible that the PCC wanted other works to be more conservative and the content more closely monitored.

The book was problematic in some regards as it provided detailed information on an extremely wide range of topics. It sparked national debate on sexual education, sexual health, and, particularly, sexual diversity as it presented homosexuality as normal. The book's final chapter, entitled "Homosexuality in Man and Woman" ("Homosexualidad en el hombre y la mujer"), discussed the importance of respect for men and women of different sexual orientations. The author asserted that 3 to 4 percent of the population were homosexual, and incorporated a full discussion of why homosexuality should be categorized within normal sexual behavior. The chapter noted that there had been various scientific theories of how homosexuality occurred, or was "spread." In particular "seduction" was noted as a common understanding of how men become homosexuals. Schnabl also explained that there had been several scientific studies on animals in an effort to determine a scientific cause of homosexuality. However he contended that there were instead various psychosocial causes of homosexuality. In addition, he noted that, for both men and women, sexual orientation could not be changed, and asserted that homosexuality was a variant of sexuality and as such could not be classified as an illness. He continued to explain that, as a result of social stigma, many homosexuals wanted to change their sexual orientation—often searching for treatments or help. Homosexual men and women, he argued, could be good parents, and compared homophobic people to Nazis. Indeed, the central thesis throughout the chapter was that homosexuals needed to be respected, as they should respect others, because under socialism everyone was afforded equal rights. Moreover, unlike the other chapters, which were written in a very detached and clinical way, the chapter was written in a very empathetic way, and focused on health and well-being. He employed medical data relating to sexually diverse persons, including information regarding mental health issues and suicides as a result of prejudice and discrimination, in order to demand respect for homosexuality and societal change. This popular book fortified the discrimination-health link that had been established earlier by the FMC. While the FMC has applied this method as a means of improving abortion rights and normalizing them, Schnabl used the same argument to promote sexual diversity rights. He similarly employed the discrimination-health link to normalize prejudiced behavior on the basis of the importance of national health.

This book was also a significant step in the incorporation of sexuality and sexual education into national debate because it presented women as sexual beings. It developed a new understanding of women, since to a large extent their sexuality had previously been ignored. Women's sexuality had been traditionally associated almost exclusively with reproductive health, which was evident in the early push for the legalization of abortions (1965) and the focus on maternal and child mortality rates. Importantly, however, the book discussed women's sexuality in the same manner in which men's sexuality was discussed—as normal human behavior.

Following the success of Schnabl's book, in 1981 another of his books, *In Defense of Love* (*En defensa del amor*), was also published, and later reprinted in 1985. While the first was more factual, and focused on educating readers about the mechanics of sexuality and sexual health, the second book discussed sexuality in society. Its central theme was that everyone had a right to a safe and satisfying sexual life, and emphasized the author's contention that love and sexuality were integral aspects of a person's life and as such needed to be better understood. As he explained, "Love and sexuality are not dangerous diseases from which we have to protect our children" (Schnabl 1981, 26). Again, Schnabl emphasized a health-based approach to normalize sexual diversity.

This book was also significant because it discussed sexuality as an important component of the national expression of socialist ideology. The author explained that sexuality was an important aspect of an individual's and of a society's development. Thus, under socialism, a person's given sexuality must be respected. For example, he noted,

> The Marxist-Leninist conception, as the scientific foundation of our socialist social system is—in its essence—a confirmation of life, and because of this it also considers sexual activity that contributes to happiness, contentment, fulfilment, satisfaction and the enrichment of man's existence to be positive. This conception is based upon the proposals and conclusions of Marx, Engels, Lenin, Bebel and others. (Schnabl 1981, 6–7)

He later used the same argument for homosexuality, noting that under socialism different sexual expressions must also be respected. He supported his point by making a comparison between the repressive capitalist societies, which viewed homosexuality as a perversion, and socialist ones, which in contrast were supposed to liberate their populations. He asserted that under socialism everyone must be considered equal, and respected—and this extended to individual sexuality.

Beyond its ideological significance, this book was also very important because it made a clear connection between sexuality and sexual health. It explained that a safe and satisfactory sexual life was important for individuals, and a vital aspect of that was sexual health. It was thus important because it allowed for a more developed and safer society—the logic being that, as sexuality is important, sexual health must be equally important. This work was extremely popular and widely read. *Mujeres* even published much of the book in small excerpts (FMC 1984b, 56–57).

It is clear that GNTES was fundamental in the book's publication. Its prologue discussed the work of GNTES, and noted the support of the FMC in particular, as well as the contributions of Álvarez Lajonchere and Krause. As was the case with its precursor, this book was also published by MINCULT. Notably, however, Schnabl's prologue also mentioned the

National Assembly's Permanent Commission On the Attention to Infancy, Youth, and the Equality of Rights of Women (Schnabl 1981). This clearly indicated the ongoing importance of this Commission, and that it was fulfilling its original aim of publishing works of significance.

The work of Brückner was also published in various books. He was a pediatrician specializing in sexuality and sexual health, and wrote three significant books that were translated in Cuba. The first two, titled *When Your Child Asks You* (*Cuando tu hijo te pregunta*) and *Before a Child is Born* (*Antes de que nazca un niño*), were published in 1979 (and later reprinted the following year) (Brückner 1980a; Brückner 1980b). The first was very instructive for parents, explaining in detail how to discuss sexual and reproductive health with children aged one to twelve, and outlined the most common questions that arise at different ages, and how they should be answered (Brückner 1980b, 27).

The book also answered questions directed at parents. One question that was asked, for example, was whether talking to one's children when they were young about sex and reproduction could have negative consequences or make them more curious. Brückner, however, explained that, if a child was mature enough to ask a question, then they were mature enough to know the answer. The book focused on developing an open and honest dialogue about sexuality, explaining that children must learn from an early age that sexually responsible behavior was important. He also posited that children with a better understanding of sexuality and reproduction would become more respectful and responsible adults (Brückner 1980b).

Brückner's second book published in Cuba was originally written in 1971 in East Germany, and later reprinted in Cuba in 1979 and 1980. The book was produced as a tool for parents and teachers to explain reproduction and sexual organs to children, aged nine to twelve. Brückner's last popular-science book published in Cuba was *Are You Now Thinking About Love?* (*¿Piensas ya en el amor?*), originally published in Cuba in 1981, with a second edition a year later, and reprinted again in 1985. This book was important because, as stated in a preliminary note,

> For the Cuban version, chapter 12 has been rewritten, and some changes and adaptations have been made to other chapters, in light of suggestions and considerations made by representatives of the National Working Group on Sexual Education, which is an adjunct of the Permanent Commission of the National Assembly. This is related to "the attention to infancy and the equality of rights held by women" and to the special revision of a commission of the Ministry of Education. (Brückner 1981)

The significance was in the fact that it was the only book that stated that it had undergone revisions (by a Cuban organization, probably from MINCULT), or any specific MINED commission. It is unclear which specific changes were undertaken; chapter 12, however, was titled "Sexual Variation and Deviations" ("Variantes y desviaciones sexuales"), and discussed homosexuality as a deviation and a problem.[7]

This book, in contrast to the work of Schnabl, was written in a homophobic manner. For example, Brückner explained,

> Certain homosexuals call attention to themselves because of their scandalous and antisocial behavior. At times some of them try to take advantage of children and adolescents, and approach them with a variety of strategies in order to satisfy their homosexual activities. (Brückner 1981, 210)

He continued to assert that any parent or teacher who saw a child apparently engaged in homosexual actions or mannerisms, or any children themselves who were aware of their problem, should seek professional and specialized help (Brückner 1981, 210).

The book's information regarding homosexuality contradicted that of Schnabl's *Man and Woman in Intimacy*. As it is very unlikely that GNTES chose to publish literature that discussed sexual diversity in this way, particularly as the group had earlier supported literature that promoted respect for diversity, it is likely that this was either the author's original work, or that it was changed in Cuba to reflect prejudicial attitudes. This could have been the result of the MINED Commission, or another contributing editing body that chose to change the work. Notably, the term "antisocial" was used throughout the section on homosexuality, suggesting that it was amended or changed in Cuba, as the term had previously been strongly, although not exclusively, associated with homosexuality throughout the first two decades of the Revolution. Nonetheless, as the term was also common in Eastern Europe for activities deemed unacceptable (but not necessarily directly counter-revolutionary), the origins of the amendments remain unclear.

Yet despite the change in attitude toward sexual diversity, the rest of the book followed a similar ideological stance to the others published. Socialism was the clear ideological framework, with a particular emphasis on the role of the state. Moreover, there was a focus on gender equality and respect.

In addition to the imported and translated works, Krause also published two books. The first was *Some Fundamental Themes in Sexual Education* (*Algunos temas fundamentales sobre educación sexual*), published in 1985. It was later expanded, with two sections added: "Sexual Education and Its Political-Ideological Nature" ("Educación sexual y su carácter político-ideológico") and "Why is Sexual Education Necessary?" ("¿Por qué la educación sexual es necesaria?"), and was reprinted in 1987, and again in 1988 (Krause 1987; 1988). A central theme throughout the work was that sexual education was required in order to have relationships based on love, consideration, solidarity, friendship, and mutual respect (Krause 1985).

Her second book, published in 1987 and reprinted in 1988, was *Sexual Education: Selected Lectures* (*Educación sexual. Selección de lecturas*). It assembled round-table answers provided by GNTES members, including Espín and Álvarez Lajonchere. In particular, the book was important because it provided direct expertise and opinions from GNTES, using their own words to discuss sexual education. It posed questions, and the corresponding reflections from the individuals were provided.

Krause's books were significant because they allowed a direct channel for the opinions of GNTES and its members to be published, providing their clear positions on various topics relating to sexuality and sexual education. Although she was technically a foreign author, Krause's books were written with a Cuban understanding of sexual education, and were among the first produced on the island, rather than being imported and translated (linguistically and culturally).

THIRD AND FOURTH FMC CONGRESSES: SEXUAL EDUCATION AND SEXUAL HEALTH, 1980–1984

Many of the specifics of the development of the national sexual education program are unrecorded, as are the details of the development of TV and radio programs. Although some of the literature has noted the significance of these programs (Krause 1987; 1988), none have offered details. For example, it is unclear when TV programs regarding sexual education began, or how many students and professionals participated in GNTES' sexual education courses and seminars. Yet analysis of the 3rd and 4th FMC Congresses is instructive, illustrating that, while some details are unavailable, the overall direction of the FMC and sexual health in Cuba throughout the 1980s can be understood. During this period GNTES became increasingly important to both the development of ProNes, and the incorporation of sexuality into the national debate, highlighting the negotiative process.

The 3rd FMC Congress was held in 1980 and attended by approximately 2,000 delegates, representing some two million *federadas* (FMC 1984a, 6; *Granma* 1977a). While the Congress was of interest for various reasons, it was particularly significant in terms of the development of sexual education and sexual health. The most notable aspect of the Congress was the Thesis entitled "Sexaul Aspects of the Ideological Struggle. The Role of Women. Ideological Topics Required to Obtain Complete Equality" ("Algunos aspectos de la lucha ideológica. Papel de la Mujer. Tareas ideológicas encaminadas al ejercicio de la plena igualdad"), of which Section Eight, "Education in the Family" ("La educación de la familia"), paid particular attention to sexual education and GNTES (FMC

1984a, 64–67). It outlined the importance of GNTES, emphasizing it as having a vital role in providing sexual education, sexual health and the development of sexually responsible citizens (FMC 1984a, 67).

The recommendations offered by the 3rd Congress were indicative of the national developments relating to sexual education. The Congress suggested that sexual education should begin at a young age, and increase in complexity and breadth of material. Moreover, it suggested that sexual education for the general populace also be increased, as its role too was important in the education of younger generations. Furthermore, the Congress recommended that publications relating to sexual education (such as literature and pamphlets) be increased in terms of production and distribution. Finally, it was also recommended that more work be done regarding sexual problems, such as sexual dysfunction. In particular, the Congress suggested that courses touching upon sexuality be developed for fields that dealt with issues surrounding sexuality, mainly those working in the medical field.

A central theme throughout the section was the incorporation of sexuality into medical care. In other words, the FMC was increasingly focusing on sexual education as an important aspect of healthcare, as it continued to employ its health-based approach. Significant references were made to sexual education being provided in medical training programs, as well as the training of psychologists and social workers. While the connection was not made explicit, the trend was clear: sexual education was linked firmly to health.

The 4th FMC Congress dramatically increased the emphasis on sexual education, sexual health, and in particular the role of GNTES. The Congress took place in 1984, with a similar number of delegates as at the 3rd Congress, and emphasized women as being responsible for educating the family. Notably, GNTES was lauded in the opening synopsis of the work of the FMC (FMC 1987, 19–20). Two Commissions from this Congress stood out as being particularly important, and illustrative of the ongoing development of national attitudes toward sexuality. The first was the "Commission 3: Questions Concerning the Integration of Women in Economic Activities" ("Comisión no. 3: Cuestiones referentes a la integración de la mujer a la vida económica"), which had a specific section on health, "Resolution Regarding Health ("Resolución sobre la salud"). It noted the importance of the *brigadistas* in continuing to engage in the provision of healthcare, particularly for women and children, and incorporated discussion about the importance of increasing sexual education. "Commission 5: Questions Concerning Women and Their Participation in Cultural, Educational and Social Life" ("Comisión no. 5: Cuestiones relativas a la mujer y su participación en la vida cultural, educacional y social") was also significant. Of particular importance was the "Resolution on Educating the Family and the Formation of New Generations" ("Resolución sobre la educación de la familia y la formación de las nuevas generaciones"). It explained that any "prejudices," "taboos" or "discrimination" that affected the development of sexually responsible citizens were unacceptable (FMC 1987, 103). The list of the final recommendations of the Congress also provided a clear emphasis on the themes of sexual education and sexual health.

The First Recommendation made by the Congress was in regard to education and referred to the family structure. It recommended that further books and pamphlets (particularly popular-science works) be created in order to assist parents when teaching the children "The Correct Sexual Education" ("la correcta educación sexual") (FMC 1987, 104).

The Second Recommendation emphasized the importance of the ongoing work of MINED, increasing its work in the field of sexual education in order to systematically introduce it at all the levels of the National Education Program, as well as at parents' meetings (FMC 1987, 106).

The Fifth Recommendation promoted the further incorporation of working relationships between significant national organizations, such as the National Union of Cuban Jurists (Unión Nacional de Juristas de Cuba) (UNJC) and FEU. Part of the recommendation included the need to assist GNTES with its research relating to, among other things, "attitudes," "relationships," and "sexuality" (FMC 1987, 108).

The Sixth Recommendation did not mention GNTES, but focused specifically on health and family planning, one section for example, stated that it: "Recommend to MINSAP that the possibility be considered of increasing specialized consultations in sexual matters for couples, family, and young people. It also recommends that special consultation facilities be established for adolescents, where they can discuss problems relating to sexuality" (FMC 1987, 109).

Finally, the Seventh Recommendation focused on the means of communication, such as television, radio, and cinema, which contributed to ideological formation. The recommendation suggested that GNTES coordinate with the FMC, MINED, MINSAP, and the UJC to increase the distribution of information regarding risks related to teenage pregnancy, STIs, and the responsible use of contraception (FMC 1987, 110).

What is clear from the Congress is that the question of sexuality had become gradually more incorporated into social justice issues, as well as issues relating to health and education. Of particular significance too was the increased importance placed on GNTES working with MINSAP; the FMC recommendations emphasized the important relationship between them.

SEXUAL DISCOURSE IN *BOHEMIA*, 1985–1989

By the late 1980s, sexual education, sexual health, and the concept of sexuality had become fully incorporated into the national debate. The emphasis placed by the FMC, and later the PCC and National Assembly on the topics had dramatically increased debate and work on these topics. An example of this was the dramatic increase (and in some cases introduction) of related discussions in the media, and print in particular.

An analysis of the popular magazine *Bohemia* is instructive, illustrating the increasing coverage of, and interest in, sexuality. For instance, the first *Bohemia* article focusing on the importance of sexual education was published in an April 1987 edition. Titled "Sexual Education: Outdated Traditions and Customs" ("Educación sexual: Tradiciones y costumbres anacrónicas"), the article asserted the need to incorporate sexuality as an integral component of education.

Similarly, the first mention of GNTES in any issue of *Bohemia* was in the June 1987 edition. The article, "Teenage Pregnancy: A fast-Moving Epidemic" ("Embarazo en la adolescencia: Epidemia de alta frecuencia"), discussed in detail the reasons for increased pregnancy rates in teenagers. The article concluded by stressing the need for better sexual health education and birth control options (*Bohemia* 1987b, 21–25). The following edition (in July 1987) published another article, "Television and Sex" ("La televisión y el sexo") (*Bohemia* 1987c, 84). The article was written by Krause (the first time her name appeared in *Bohemia,* where she is described as the *coordinadora* of GNTES), who discussed sexual education as an integral aspect of education. She explained in detail the need for sexual health to be taught to adolescents.

The presence of these articles in a popular magazine is indicative of the shift in the understanding of sexuality in Cuba. Sexual education and sexual health were clearly no longer aims solely of the FMC, GNTES, or the government, but also represent the aims of society, as the ongoing national debate on sexuality rapidly evolved.

The most important contribution made by the FMC was the employment of a health-based approach and establishing the discrimination-health link, which underpinned many women's sexual health issues. In addition to establishing an approach that would continue to be used in future endeavors, this highlighted the Revolution's capacity for change through a negotiative process. From this closer examination, the significance of the FMC's role becomes clear, providing another piece to the puzzling process of the island's normalization of sexual diversity.

By the late 1980s, the importance of sexual education and sexual health, and GNTES in particular, was clear. In 1988 the Minister of Health signed a resolution to change GNTES into CENESEX, and the following year it was officially founded as a MINSAP center (Castro Espín 2013 [Interview]). The importance of this is threefold. First, it shows that the government believed that sexual education was integral to national development, re-establishing GNTES as an official Center dedicated to sexual education. Second, this is also demonstrative of the importance that sexuality was taking on—as a respected branch of health and healthcare, illustrating the importance placed on sexual education as a means of achieving sexual health. Finally, it illustrates the capacity of the Revolution to evolve and adapt to contemporary needs. This change in 1989 would later prove vital for the normalization of sexual diversity, as CENESEX would receive international acclaim, and fame.

NOTES

1. For further examples, see Bengelsdorf 1997; Montero Maldonado 1996; FMC 1996; Farnós Morejón et al. 1982; Ortega Guzmán 1996; Lutjens 1995; De la Cruz 1980; Fuentes 1978; González Plasencia 1996; *Granma* 1972; *Granma* 1977b; Salva 1979a, 1979b, 1979c, 1980; Salva et al. 1980.
2. For further examples, see Larguía 1973; CAME 1981; Marilley 1996; Ring 1985; Brown 1988, 461; Baksh-Soodeen 1998; Lavrin 1998; Mohanty 1991; Narayan 1997; Sandoval 1991.
3. Carolina Aguilar Ayerra is one of the initial founders of the FMC, working closely with Yolanda Ferrer and Vilma Espín, among others. As a trained journalist, she worked for the FMC in publishing, editing dozens of books and hundreds of magazines, and remains heavily involved in the organization.
4. Examples of the *Hablemos fracamente* section include, de la Cuesta Freijomil 1997; Ravelo 2007a; Ravelo 2007b; Ravelo 1999.
5. Until now it was believed that the year the group was formed was generally 1977. For example, researchers including Hamilton (2012, 36), Smith and Padula (1996, 174) and Lumsden (1996, 78) noted 1977, while Krause-Fuchs (2007, 112) noted 1976 as year of GNTES was founded.
6. The National Assembly's Permanent Commission On the Attention to Infancy, Youth, and the Equality of Rights of Women was referred to in Spanish as either la Comisión Permanente de la Asamblea Nacional del Poder Popular "Sobre la atención a la infancia y la igualdad de derechos de la mujer," or the "Comisión Permanente para la Atención a la Infancia, la Juventud, y la Igualdad de Derechos de la Mujer" (*Granma* 1977c).
7. Despite significant effort, attempts to locate the original German edition were unfortunately unsuccessful. It remains unclear what changes were made in the Cuban edited edition.

THREE

Combating Discrimination

The National Center of Sexual Education (CENESEX), 1990–2015

The 1990s were some of the most economically difficult years for revolutionary Cuba. With the collapse of the Soviet Union and ongoing tensions with the United States, the country faced considerable economic challenges. Yet, while Cuba was struggling economically and in the process of developing new economic strategies, dramatic social changes began to emerge. One such change was that of attitudes toward sexual diversity.

CENESEX was established in 1989 under MINSAP, largely because, while GNTES had significantly developed sexual education and sexual health, it was clear that a new organization was required to meet the changing demands of Cuban society. A need for improved sexual education was evident, as the government noted ongoing related problems, including high STIs and abortion rates. Although GNTES had successfully incorporated sexuality into national debate, the new challenges facing Cuba made a more comprehensive approach necessary.

THE EVOLUTION OF CENESEX

CENESEX in the 1990s

Very little is known about CENESEX in the 1990s. Besides the lack of real research, one must also consider the substantial economic pressures on publishing. Thus there is almost no information regarding the Center during that period to be found in international publications, with the limited publications produced by the Center being available only in its archives.

In order to understand CENESEX at the time, it is important to remember that until 1989 it had been led solely by the FMC, and in particular by Espín and Álvarez Lajonchere (and to some degree by Krause until 1990). Following its transfer to MINSAP, the FMC and those who had been working for GNTES maintained control over the Center and its projects. Álvarez Lajonchere worked as the primary director, with others taking over when he was engaged in projects elsewhere. In the 1990s, the Center consolidated its aims and education strategies, rooted in the health and well-being of the island.

In some ways the 1990s (usually referred to as the Special Period) worked to the benefit of the Center, largely allowing it to develop without considerable influence from MINSAP, other ministries, or the National Assembly. During this economically devastating period, the government continued to invest heavily in healthcare and education. Moreover, as a result of the pressures, the extensive economic crisis allowed (and in some cases encouraged) centers and ministries to work with greater autonomy. For CENESEX, this meant that, as a part of MINSAP and with a focus on education, it continued to be a priority, and was able to develop with notable independence. This autonomy was in some ways furthered by the Center working with international bodies such as the UN and some NGOs, from which it received financial support for publications and family planning programs.

Throughout the 1990s, the Center diversified its interests and aims. While GNTES primarily focused on research and developing ProNes, CENESEX expanded its initiatives and goals to include an increased emphasis on research into the concepts of gender and sexuality, as well as a number of audio-visual media initiatives, postgraduate courses, and awareness-building. In 1994, for example, following what the current director referred to as an "experience" in Pilón, Granma province, the Center incorporated community development programs into its objectives (Castro Espín 2013 [Interview]).

CENESEX sought and received funding from international bodies, with the most significant contributions coming from the UN, for projects relating to sexual education and family planning. As a result of the UN funding, the Center was able to dramatically increase the breadth of its work. For example, in 1993 it was able to establish the "Cátedras" of Sexology and Education (Cátedras de Sexología y Educación) and for Sexual Education (Cátedras para la Educación Sexual) in various medical institutes, as well as the National School of Public Health (Escuela Nacional de Salud Pública) (Castro Espín 2013 [Interview]; CENESEX 2012a). It is significant that they work within the healthcare field, and especially the area of health training. Clearly, from the early 1990s, CENESEX viewed medical training, and the practice of medicine, as an area in which the importance of sexuality and sexual education needed to be emphasized.

In the early 1990s, CENESEX also created a new newspaper column focused on sexuality in the newspaper geared toward young people, *Juventud Rebelde*. Titled *Sexo Sentido*, it provided an open area for national debate, questions, advice, and the dissemination of information. The column was written by experts specializing in different areas of sexuality, gender studies and health, and continued to increase the number of articles on sexual diversity, particularly from 2008.

As a result of external funding, in 1994 the Center began producing its research journal, *Sexology and Society* (*Sexología y Sociedad*). The journal was particularly important as a means of distributing information because it discussed research conducted both in Cuba and abroad, incorporating the works of other international studies and specialists. Moreover, a letter from the editor that was a feature of the journal functioned as an editorial on contemporary issues relating to sexuality in Cuba. While, in 1994, there was only one issue of the journal published, by the end of the 1990s it was published quarterly, and gradually increased in distribution and prestige.

By the mid-1990s, CENESEX had established itself as a significant force within MINSAP. The Center was collaborating with several ministries and organizations on various projects relating to sexuality, and continued to increase its role in Cuba and internationally. In 1997, for example, Cuba hosted the Latin American Congress of Sexual Education, which later became the Latin American Congress of Sexology and Sexual Education (Congreso Latinoamericano de Sexología y Educación Sexual) (CLASES). The Center continued to participate in and host international meetings and conferences in the area. It developed its own identity, with a considerable emphasis on research and various national programs that sought to increase the country's understanding of sexuality.

In the early 1990s, Castro Espín was appointed to the Center. A self-described socialist, she graduated from the University of Havana with a degree in Child Psychology. She originally wanted to work as a presenter on a children's educational TV show, and it was largely at the urging of Álvarez Lajonchere, a family friend who had also done sexual education presentations in her school when she was a girl, that she began working for CENESEX (Castro Espín 2013 [Interview]). While neither she nor her familial ties to the government were discussed in the national or international media at the time, she would later become a significant international figure. Castro Espín received her PhD in Sociology in 2015. Her thesis focused on issues facing transgender Cubans, a topic she had been championing for years. While often compared to her father outside of Cuba, it is clear that she is her mother's daughter in demeanor, charisma, and physical appearance. With her compassion and direct style of leadership, it is evident at the Center that she is highly respected as the Director and is well regarded by the staff and patients alike.

Throughout the 1990s, the Center's main strategy was the discrimination-health link. Through its various education programs, it sought to demonstrate the considerable health-related risks associated to sexuality-based discrimination. For example, an unpublished CENESEX report on the national sexual education program from the early to mid-1990s[1] illustrates this strategy. The report included various exercises for students. In one, students were instructed to "imagine that you are just phoned by a very close friend. He tells you that he believes he is homosexual, which he finds very difficult to accept, and as a result is thinking of committing suicide. However the phones go out mid-conversation and will not be back on until the following day." The student was then instructed to write a twenty-word telegram, responding to his friend (Centro Nacional de Educación Sexual, n.d.).

This early emphasis on combating discrimination toward sexuality through a health-based approach was critical, as it laid the groundwork for the incorporation of the normalization of sexual diversity, as a basic concept, into the Center's main aims some years later.

CENESEX, 2000–2015

Between 2003 and 2004, the focus of CENESEX shifted to emphasize respect for sexual diversity, and the Center increased its work significantly in the area. Its website started publishing more data on the topic, while at the same time more related research was being undertaken, campaigns were being developed, and events were increasingly held. Similarly, specific workshops, panels, and courses on the theme of sexual diversity were established. Rather than maintaining the previous focus on the issue of men who have sex with men, the Center now increased its interests to incorporate various needs regarding sexual diversity.

One might argue that this dramatic shift was the result of the appointment to the Center's staff of two activists, a physician and a specialist in public relations, who suggested focusing more specifically on sexual diversity and related rights. Similarly, it could be argued that it was a personal choice of the director, who has noted in various articles and interviews that in 2004 the Center had received requests regarding care for transgender persons, an area that led to a greater focus on sexual diversity. This could certainly be viewed as a natural progression, as the Center housed numerous specialists who focused on the psychological, physical, and social issues related to transgender persons. Instead, analysis of the evolution of the Center's earlier work suggests that the shift was the result of various corresponding factors, and was a response to a national need and demand for increased attention to sexual diversity.

CENESEX began developing its programs regarding sexual diversity in the late 1980s and early 1990s, following the emergence of HIV/AIDS and the subsequent increase in infection rates. The Cuban government had an aggressive prevention and treatment program, but in 2000 CENESEX began working on MINSAP's preventive project titled Men who Have Sex with Men (Hombres que tienen sexo con hombres) focused primarily on bisexual and homosexual men, the groups statistically most affected by HIV/AIDS.

Meanwhile, the topic of sexuality and the field of sexology were increasingly a priority within the Center, and representatives attended the 2003 World Congress on Sexology. Sexuality was being developed as a legitimate area of academic study, as well as a health indicator (CENESEX 2005). By 2004, the social need to develop work on sexual diversity became apparent, as the topic was increasingly broached in national debate and academic fora. As Marta María Ramírez[2] (2013 [Interview]), CENESEX Social Communication Representative, explained "It was established to fill the demand and need of the people." This is important as it indicated the ongoing and intensifying national debate on sexuality, and the public demand for further information regarding sexual diversity. Moreover, it indicated that government officials and ministries were open to debate, as well as providing the requested information.

In 2007, CENESEX participated for the first time in celebrations of the International Day Against Homophobia (in Cuba the *Jornada contra la homofobia*). Since 2008, the Center has continued to increase its emphasis on sexual diversity, and particularly the incorporation of this issue into ProNes and its curricula. Through workshops, courses, parties, book fairs, art shows, and literature, the Center has (beginning in 2004 and emphasized since 2008) continued to fully incorporate sexual diversity into its work and central aims.

The initial steps that it undertook to promote sexual health and respect for sexual diversity were seen clearly in a series of campaigns. Since 2004, the Center has established and developed various campaigns on sexual health, with an emphasis on condom use, and particularly HIV/AIDS prevention. They are promoted in diverse formats, including posters, pamphlets, advertisements in the Center's published work, and also discussed at various CENESEX events. For example one campaign, established in 2006, titled How Do I Show You That I Love you? (*¿Cómo demuestro que te amo?*), with the tagline of "Enjoy Life, Avoid AIDS" ("Disfruta la vida, evita el SIDA"), focuses on HIV/AIDS prevention through the use of condoms, and engaging in safe sex only. Significantly, the posters promoting the campaign are made with both male and female figures, suggesting the shared responsibility for condom use, rather than the sole responsibility of males.

Among the most significant campaigns is Diversity is Natural (*La diversidad es natural*), established in 2009. It promotes social and juridical sexual diversity rights, as well as a general respect for diverse sexual orientations. There are four posters promoting the campaign, including one showing two women's panties hanging on a line to dry, as well as another with two men's boxer shorts and a similar theme expressed by having a poster with two men's shaving brushes, and two tea cups marked with lipstick, each with the slogan "Two of the Same Also Make a Couple" ("Dos iguales también hacen pareja"). This campaign is aimed largely at adolescents; as Castro Espín notes, "it is from here that the future professionals and directors of Cuban society will emerge" (Grogg 2009).

Another campaign, and a joint effort between CENESEX and the Cuban Institute of Cinematographic Arts and Industry (Instituto Cubano del Arte e Industria Cinematográficos) (ICAIC), is *Cine Club Diferente.* It was established in 2008, during the *Jornada Contra la Homofobia,* and convenes once a month (Jorge 2009; Puentes 2012). It can best be understood as a monthly event, rather than a campaign, as each session consists of watching a film that focuses on themes of sexuality or sexual diversity, followed by a debate where specialists from the Center, as well as those from other institutions, and the general populace participate. Afterwards, questions regarding sexual diversity rights are raised and discussed from different points of view and experiences. Although some Cuban films have been featured (such as Green Green) (*Verde Verde*), the films presented are usually international (including from, among others, Great Britain, the United States, Japan, Argentina and Korea), such as *Maurice, Habitación en Roma, XXY, Boys don't Cry, The Bubble, Trembling before G-d, What Makes a Family,* and *Bent* (WebCENESEX 2012a; WebCENESEX 2012b; Pineda Barnet 2012).

Other CENESEX campaigns include The Entire World Is Important (*Todo el mundo cuenta*), It's Your World (*Es tu mundo*), and Communication and Education (*Comunicacional y Educativa*), and focus primarily on young people (Labacena Romero and Felipe González 2011). *Comunicacional y Educativa,* for example, was established in 2011, and focuses on the development of institutional programs relating to sexual diversity and gender by young sexual health promoters. Through this campaign, university students in areas such as the Medical Sciences, Pedagogy, Cultural Studies, and Sport Sciences have received sensitivity and sexual health training from their peers. The central theme of these campaigns is the concept of young people training other young people; the idea is that participants will be more receptive if the information is coming from their peers. The campaigns have been effective in raising awareness of issues relating to sexual diversity and sexual health, and have continued to increase in breadth and numbers of participants.

In addition to its academic, activist, and research initiatives, the Center houses several medical professionals such as doctors and nurses, psychologists, psychiatrists, and therapists who regularly see patients for sexuality-related issues. The medical care given is largely primary care, with more advanced care offered elsewhere. Although CENESEX is rarely, if ever, discussed in the international fora as a medical facility, it is important to remember that, despite being formally an educational institution, it is a MINSAP center.

The CENESEX building and the numbers of specialists have also increased dramatically. In the early 2000s, when Castro Espín became director, the Center was moved to a new and larger location in Vedado, Havana. While GNTES was made up of only a few specialists, by 2013 there were over sixty staff members at CENESEX, including public relations specialists, journalists, sexologists, psychologists, nurses, doctors, researchers and academics, as well as a lawyer and a librarian. The work of the Center also increased to incorporate various areas of sexual health, such as domestic violence. Moreover, various Masters and Diploma courses have been offered since the early 2000s, as the Center promotes and assists in academic studies on themes relating to gender and sexuality.

Those employed at the Center endeavor to create an accepting and respectful environment, and they are extremely varied—from specialties, genders, sexual orientations, ages, and responsibilities. As a clear indication of the Center's commitment to respect for diversity, for example, the bathrooms are unmarked, with no sign of the female and male caricatures.

THE STRUCTURE OF CENESEX AND PRONES CURRICULA, 1990–2015

By the mid-1990s, like its predecessor GNTES, CENESEX was still responsible for carrying out the National Assembly's Permanent Commission On the Attention to Infancy, Youth and the Equality of Rights of Women, and continued to do so through education, building on the FMC's work, and particularly the discrimination-health link.

The organizational structure of ProNes, developed through national debate, was complex. Known as the Line of Work (*línea de trabajo*), the makeup consisted of several levels of authority, each with specific responsibilities, from the National Assembly down to local leaders and individuals who the Center believed had a significant capacity to carry out its work. The Center, working below the National Assembly and officially as an entity of MINSAP, has a Council of Representatives, made up of representatives from MINED, MINSAP, FMC, and other political and student organizations, such as FEU (Flórez Madan 1994, 24). The Council of Representatives had a reciprocal relationship, as CENESEX would make recommendations, while also receiving suggestions for the efficacy of its programs.

CENESEX and the members of the Council would then implement decisions or programs (particularly relating to training in areas regarding education and health) through the Provincial Commissions on Sexual Education, which would in turn continue to implement them in the Municipal Commissions on Sexual Education. In total, by 1994 there were 169 Municipal Commissions (one in each municipality), which would then introduce the necessary instructions or information to communities. Responsibility for the information would pass to what were referred to as the "agents for change" (*agentes de cambio*), including local FMC leaders, leaders of youth groups, or anyone with a significant role within the community (Flórez Madan 1994, 24).

Each Provincial and Municipal Commission of Sexual Education maintained a multidisciplinary approach, although each focused specifically on the needs of a given area. This could include the question of abortion or STI rates that were higher than the national average, or greater rates of teenage pregnancy. If a particular need was noted, each Commission would adjust its own program in order to meet it. Moreover, the Commissions functioned as the local representation of CENESEX, maintaining the Center's presence and influence across the country.

The Center sought to implement and develop its responsibilities under the Line of Work through four main avenues including training, research, increased media and audio-visual presence, and sexual therapy. The most important component of this was training, as the Center advised on what to include in the university curricula in the fields of education and health, as well as those in schools and daycare centers. Workshops, seminars, courses on sexual education and efforts to work out the best means to implement these goals were also developed for professionals, such as doctors, psychologists, professors, teachers, as well as social and community development workers. The training stressed the importance of participation and community development, suggesting that one was more likely to learn, as well as pass on the information, if one felt involved in the process. The idea was that change and improvements are optimized through debate, rather than occurring through efforts directed by the government through a top-down approach.

The National Sexual Education Program, ProNes, was comprehensive and extensive. Through the Line of Work, ProNes can be understood as having been implemented through two spheres: the formal and informal. The formal sphere of this program focused on educational institutions, including higher-education levels, such as medical faculties, and educational institutions (including teaching institutions). In addition, it included the implementation of the ProNes curricula in daycares, preschools, primary, junior high and high school levels, as well as polytechnic institutions. While the ProNes curricula were not standardized across each level, they were similar and based on the needs of a specific region.

The informal sphere through which ProNes was implemented was extensive and included the various areas in which sexual education was taught by representatives outside of the formal education system. Information was provided by the "agents of change," who worked through the Provincial and Municipal Sexual Education Commissions to distribute the information widely. Beginning in the early 1990s, young people known as "health promoters" were also trained, with the aim of sharing the information among their peers (McPherson Sayú 1995, 7–9; Rodríguez Lauzurique 1994, 30–31).

Beginning in 1996, a standardized sexual education program was implemented in the national school system, in which children would continue to learn about sexuality (Castro Espín, 2013 [Interview]; Vázquez Seijido[3] 2013 [Interview]). There is little data on the specifics of the program, but it included annual comprehensive courses, on which the students were tested, and presentations by specialists. As Flórez Madan (1994, 27) explained, "We professionals of CENESEX have the duty to remain up to date with our education and approach, and especially to channel the science of sexology to support the true potential and capacity of human beings and ensuring that there is no sexual discrimination."

Studies have shown that Cuban children and young people believe that they have a good sexual education program. One study found that 81.6 percent of junior high school students and 83.3 percent of high school students felt that they were receiving a good sexual education. The same study also suggested that 73.5 percent of junior high school students and 77.7 percent of high school students talked to their parents about sex and related issues (Ravelo 2005, 175–76). Yet specialists believed that the sexual education program in schools, as well as in general, must continue to improve, as there were ongoing problems, especially high rates of STIs, teenage pregnancies, and abortion (López Nodarse 1994, 32–33; Pantaleón 2009).

In 2012 CENESEX, along with various ministries, began developing the next stage in the sexual education program, the National Program of Sexual Education and Sexual Health (Programa Nacional de Educación y Salud Sexual)—or ProNess. It was believed that, due to changes in the Center's emphasis on sexual diversity, changes throughout the entire curricula were also needed (Vázquez Seijido 2013 [Interview]). The new ProNess, implemented between 2013 and 2014, incorporated sexual diversity into the education and health curricula, and aimed to continue to promote comprehensive sexual education and sexual healthcare services. The curricula in schools, for example, have been re-written to teach about sexual diversity, and in particular to teach children and young people about the sexual health needs of sexually diverse groups. The health-based approach is employed throughout the curricula, as the material states clearly that discrimination is harmful to health for all sexual orientations.

The idea was that, since Cuba's sexually diverse population represents a significant amount of the country's population, it is the responsibility of the government, and in particular MINSAP and MINED via CENESEX, to address their specific sexual education and sexual health needs. However, there are other contemporary issues that some believe should be incorporated into ProNess, including domestic violence, and discrimination on the basis of religion or race, among others, as one's health and well-being (sexual and otherwise) are also dependent on these (Alfonso Rodríguez 2007; Chávez Negrín 2011; Aguilera Ribeaux 2001).

NETWORKS

An important method used by CENESEX to distribute information, increase national debate, as well as conduct research, are networks, known as Community Social Networks (*Redes Sociales Comunitarias*). There are five networks, each focusing on a different group: Women, Men, Youth, Transgender and Jurist. Members of the different groups participate within the other networks, although each maintains its specific focus. They are community-based social networks, based on specific groups, through which the Center engages with the general population. While called networks by the Center, they can be best understood as a system of channels through which members can engage with the population of a given community in order to promote understanding and respect for sexual diversity. Employing a participatory framework as a means of distributing information, training, awareness-building, and conducting research, as well as assisting the Center with various events, they have continued to be an important component of CENESEX and its aims.

The concept of the networks developed from 2003, although they were not formally established as CENESEX networks until 2011 when the demand for an increased CENESEX presence throughout the island was evident and much of the groundwork for normalization had already been laid. While some were established organically outside the Center, and later became more integrated into CENESEX, others were the result of the Center's specific initiatives. Nonetheless, they served to fill a growing need for information regarding sexual diversity, and function as a considerable means of engaging the population in the public debate over sexual diversity by increasing awareness. As Roque Guerra (2013b) explains, "The establishment of social networks consists of activists for sexual rights as outlined by CENESEX. Their focus, which is on human rights, based upon principles of equality, a rejection of discrimination, and upon human dignity and solidarity, contributed to promote the inherent right to sexual identity from an institutional framework." An analysis of these networks is important in order to understand the extent of their work.

Men's Network: Red Humanidad por la Diversidad (HxD)

> "We must carry on"
>
> —Dr. Pedro Pablo Valle Artiz,[4] the former Men's Network Coordinator, 2013 [Interview]

The Men's Network, created in November 2011, has evolved from a small CENESEX group to become an important division of the Center's efforts to normalize sexual diversity. It originated from a group of CENESEX collaborators who looked at themes regarding human rights and sexual rights. Later, based on this experience, the group decided to establish Men for Diversity (*Hombres por la Diversidad*), which in 2013 changed its name to Humanity for Diversity (*Humanidad por la Diversidad*) to be more inclusive (Vázquez Seijido 2014). While it was originally meant specifically for men (homosexual, bisexual or heterosexual), the group gradually found that others wanted to join, often the mothers or friends of a member in order to show support and learn about sexual diversity. By 2013, there were several women (including lesbians) and one transgender person involved, as the diversity of the Network's participants continued to increase (Valle Artiz 2013 [Interview]).

The Men's Network meets at the Center twice a month, on the evening of every second and fourth Friday. The first meeting largely focuses on a theme on which the group will work. This could include, for example, inviting a professional from outside the Center to discuss a theme regarding sexual health, or sexual diversity, or the struggle against violence. By contrast, the second meeting could focus on anything deemed important, such as one of the Center's campaigns, holding a discussion, or talking about individual experiences. As is the case with the Center's aims, the Network works on consciousness-raising and training in an effort to normalize sexual diversity (Valle Artiz 2013 [Interview]; CENESEX 2014e).

In terms of training and consciousness-raising, the primary method employed is *cara a cara*, or face-to-face training, whereby members talk about their experiences related to sexual diversity. This could be done at the Center, or in the community, for example, through talking to co-workers. The aim of this method is to personalize the effects of homophobia and discrimination against sexual diversity. This is carried out in small groups or pairs, in order to create a more equitable relationship between the participants and to promote discussion. Significantly, the Men's Network is the only semi-open one, accepting members who did not necessarily choose to be there. At times, people are recommended to attend meetings by a member of the health service, and often by one of the Center's specialists. For example, this could include a family member of a person who has just identified himself as homosexual, and could benefit from some awareness-building training.

In addition to training, the Network works extensively with and within CENESEX, providing assistance as well as participating in the Center's activities and campaigns. These include the celebrations for the International Day Against Homophobia (*Jornada Contra la Homofobia*), movie clubs, activities related to ending violence against women, and the Center's extensive work regarding HIV/AIDS prevention. Moreover, the Men's Network participates in the training of health promoters, works on sexual health galas, participates with other Networks, and its members are often representatives on panels at various events promoting sexual health. In other words, it can be understood as working, in one way or another, in various areas of CENESEX's sexual diversity and sexual health-related efforts (CENESEX 2014e).

The Network is based in Havana, but works with, and advises, other groups across the country, and has gradually been increasing its national influence. The Men's Network has worked with a group in Cienfuegos on awareness-building training, as well as working with a group in Santiago de Cuba, Men Against Homophobia (*Hombres Contra la Homofobia*). Despite not being specifically Men's Network initiatives, these, and similar efforts, work via CENESEX and the Network, and are increasing in size and regularity across the island (Valle Artiz 2013 [Interview]).

The Men's Network has been effective in its aims, and in particular has done considerable work in consciousness-raising. Yet significant challenges remain, as it seeks to increase the breadth of its work and numbers of participants. An ongoing issue, for example, is the stigmatization of members, who are at times discriminated against for attending the meetings, and as a result maintaining or increasing numbers of participants can be difficult. Additionally, as its work is based in Havana, it continues to seek a presence in a greater number of provinces, and with larger numbers of members and participants.

Youth Network: Red de jóvenes por la salud y los derechos sexuales

> "Who are you to tolerate me? Who are you to accept me? *Respect* me."
> —Yasmany Díaz Figueroa,[5] former Youth Network Coordinator, 2013 [Interview]

The Youth Network was established in February 2012, with the aim of promoting sexual health and respect for sexual diversity. It was originally established by FEU, with members from a range of university courses, but following increased interest, it expanded to become an inclusive youth group, with members from various socioeconomic statuses, sexual orientations, religions, and educational levels.

Its principal aim is to promote sexual health and improve sexual diversity rights among young people. In particular it focuses on three elements: the promotion of sexual health, education, and social rights. The fundamental idea of the Network is that young people have the capacity to create significant change, as they will eventually be taking over leadership roles, in both professional and community capacities, and will continue to influence the following generations. Moreover, it is believed that, as a significant percentage of the population, they can continue to encourage macro and micro change within society (CENESEX 2014a).

Its central approach is the establishment and development of debate. Communication, it is believed, is a key component in the normalization of sexual diversity, promotion of rights, and attention to sexual health. Specifically, the Network works on training and consciousness-raising (such as training members how to effectively discuss prejudice and discrimination), as well as providing research on various CENESEX campaigns to analyze their efficacy, and seek improvements. Much of this is accomplished through ongoing workshops, public debates, seminars, and meetings with the Center's specialists. It is also deeply involved with various mass organizations such as FEU and UJC, as well as CENESEX programs and campaigns. For example, one of its primary campaigns is titled Its Your World (*Es tu mundo*), where the tagline is "Only You can Protect it" ("Sólo tú puedes protegerlo"). It focuses on the prevention of STIs, and HIV/AIDS in particular, with the central theme being personal responsibility. The belief is that, while the world is big and there are many factors that cannot be controlled, by contrast an individual's world—or life—is their own, and they are in control of it. They promote the need for condom use and personal responsibility regarding sexual health (Díaz Figueroa 2013 [Interview]).

In addition, the Youth Network works with CENESEX specialists to produce and distribute literature, in particular educational material, for various programs, campaigns, and coordinated efforts. They have participated, for example, in the production of material on sexual orientation, sexual diversity rights, sexual health, and HIV/AIDS prevention. The literature is written to be accessible, as the material is often read by people of different ages and educational backgrounds. They are produced with drawings, cartoons, and colors, to look more approachable to potential readers. Additionally, there is invariably content on sexual diversity, focusing on the importance of respect.

As the internet is not readily accessible in Cuba, the Youth Network uses Cuba's particular social communication channels to distribute literature and gain membership. Literature is spread by individuals (either professionals working for the Center, members of the Network, or those attending conferences and meetings across the country) who distribute the material. Young people read the material and distribute it to friends across the country. This method is not unlike that used to distribute the information in the popular-science books of the late 1970s and early 1980s. It is not a new system of disseminating information, but has been very effective. A similar method is used to communicate events or meetings. This largely includes word-of-mouth, using what Díaz Figueroa (2013 [Interview]) called "Cuba's built-in communication network." In this respect, the lack of internet has not proven to be detrimental to the work of the Network.

As of January 2013, there were some 300 members across Havana, Cienfuegos, Santiago and Sancti Spiritus, and it is being expanded to Villa Clara. Díaz Figueroa continued to explain that, "300 participants means 300 families, 300 neighborhoods, all working to change culture and prejudice." Although the newest of the Networks, the number of participants have been slowly increasing and along with it, its capacity to change attitudes toward sexual diversity.

Women's Network: Red de mujeres lesbianas y bisexuales

> "The Network is a community-based group of/for lesbian and bisexual women, in particular dealing with the health of the lesbian and bisexual community."
>
> —Dr. Ada Caridad Alfonso Rodríguez,[6] Women's Network Coordinator, 2013 [Interview]

The Women's Network was founded and developed with the principal aims of incorporating women, particularly of diverse sexual orientations, more fully into the healthcare system, as well as contributing to the normalization of sexual diversity across the island. The Network developed outside the Center in Santiago de Cuba in the early 2000s and has since increased its work across the island. Now located in CENESEX, the Network continues to evolve, working for the needs of women, with an emphasis on health, well-being and social rights (Alfonso Rodríguez 2013 [Interview]).

Its history is complex, with various stages in its development before it was eventually established to consolidate three separate women's groups that were focusing on health and sexual diversity—Las Isabelas, Oremi, and Fénix. According to journalist Dalia Acosta, the first group, Las Isabelas, was originally established in the early 1990s in Santiago de Cuba, although CENESEX would not become involved until the early 2000s (Acosta 2010b). Ada Caridad Alfonso Rodríguez, Coordinator of the Women's Network and former interim director of CENESEX explained, however, that the origins and development of the network were somewhat more complicated.

In 2003, a group of women from Santiago de Cuba who had been struggling for some time with problems regarding sexual diversity, wrote to CENESEX inquiring about issues related specifically to the health and well-being of lesbian and bisexual women, as well as general problems regarding communication. Some women were having difficulties with their families and friends, unsure of how to inform them that they were lesbians. Others were uncomfortable with having sexual feelings for other women, or did not know how to have sexual intercourse with a member of the same sex. As a result, CENESEX sent two specialists (with experience in gender studies and women's health) to Santiago to speak with the women and research their specific needs and issues. They also brought with them a considerable amount of CENESEX's published educational material, such as copies of *Sexología y Sociedad*, to contribute to the group's education (Alfonso Rodríguez 2013 [Interview]).

As a result of efforts made by the Provincial and Municipal Sexual Education Commissions, local efforts to increase education for women on sexuality were already being carried out in the region. For example, courses in a municipality of the city, focusing on women's sexual health, had been going on for some time. Yet in terms of the specific needs of lesbian and bisexual women, as well as the availability of information for those providing their medical care, some problems remained. The CENESEX specialists began identifying the specific needs and concerns of the area's sexually diverse female population. The main issues faced by the women, apart from prejudice, were health-related—physical and psychological. They found that this was largely a result of the medical system being unprepared to deal with sexual diversity; some women were uncomfortable with medical professionals using invasive equipment, as they had never had heterosexual sex and the medical procedures were painful or uncomfortable. Moreover, due to fear of prejudice and misunderstanding, many women did not want to tell their doctors of their sexual orientation or sexual activity, leaving a major aspect of their health ignored. For example, a common health and mental health issue included drug and alcohol addiction, as a result of depression, or as a means of overcoming anxiety to feel more confident when seeking sexual partners. Moreover, it was uncommon for medical professionals at the time to inquire about sex lives or the sexual orientation of patients as a diagnostic tool, leaving many women untreated.

Following research and analysis conducted by the CENESEX specialists, they began workshops dealing with these topics to support the healthy development of the members' self-esteem, and promote more positive ways of discussing their sexuality and related problems with others, such as family and friends. In addition, the improvement and development of self-esteem was considered particularly important due to women's often subordinate role in society. Over time, the breadth of the topics discussed and promoted increased, as well as membership. The group developed from a small number of women who were apprehensive about meeting in public, because of the prejudice they might face, to working with women across the region, ultimately becoming known as Las Isabelas.

Following the work in Santiago with Las Isabelas, a second women's group was founded in 2004 in Havana, named Oremi. It was composed largely of CENESEX specialists and their contacts, dealing mainly with issues relating to sexual diversity and sexual health. A group named Fénix was later established in 2008 in Cienfuegos with similar aims. Between the three groups, workshops were conducted across several of the country's provinces, including Granma and Sancti Spiritus. By 2011, the groups were working collaboratively, and in 2012 CENESEX consolidated them into the Women's Network (Acosta 2010b).

The main group is in Havana, meeting one or two Fridays a month to engage in a variety of activities such as reading poetry on women's sexuality, as well as attending debates and lectures, and watching and discussing films. From the beginning, the Women's Network gradually increased its focus on bringing attention to women's sexuality in the medical field, with an emphasis on training medical professionals about women's specific needs. For example, in the last few years, a twenty-five-credit course on sexual diversity was organized with the Medical University, which aimed to train medical professionals to learn how to talk about sexual diversity and related health issues. Along with working generally with the Center's campaigns and anti-discrimination efforts, the Women's Network also developed and participated in a variety of workshops and courses, discussing women's specific health needs in terms of sexuality, and training health promoters. For example, the program Appreciative Initiative (*Iniciativa Apreciativa*), was developed to try to identify a group or community's specific needs and to seek solutions, as well as spread any related important information or successes (CENESEX 2014c).

The Women's Network can now be understood as a community-based participatory group of and for lesbian and bisexual women, dealing particularly with health issues relating to sexual diversity. It works closely with the other Networks, and represents one of the Center's nationwide ProNess strategies focused specifically on women's sexual health needs. The Network conducts ongoing research and training, utilizing Cuba's medical and educational systems to promote the health needs of sexually diverse women.

Transgender Network: Red de personas trangénero (Trans Cuba)

> "There can be political change, but not public change."
> —Rosa Mayra Rodríguez Lauzurique,[7] Transgender Network Coordinator 2013 [Interview]

The Transgender Network developed largely within the Center as a response to a growing need for further support for Cuba's transgender community. While it could be argued it dates back to GNTES's Multidisciplinary Group, in effect a shift occurred in the early 2000s, which necessitated a national network specifically for the needs of transgender persons. Although it was not classified as one of the five Networks until 2012, in 2003–2004 the Center increased its work with the transgender community, and gradually developed a Network with the intention of increasing support for them and decreasing discrimination (Rodríguez Lauzurique 2013 [Interview]).

The primary aims of the Transgender Network include the prevention of STIs (particularly HIV/AIDS), support, training, and consciousness-raising. The prevention aspect of the Network is largely carried out by health promoters and specialists trained by the Network, who participate in workshops and training sessions with the aim of normalizing transgender needs and persons. The Network also assists in the development of related CENESEX publications, such as books that outline specifically how to hold a workshop or training session for health promoters, or specifically for a meeting with transgender persons. In addition, it works to increase the visibility of transgender citizens, from transvestites to transsexuals, while participating in specific CENESEX events and initiatives. For example, members often give talks, participate in debates, or are invited onto panels to discuss their lives and particular challenges (CENESEX 2014d).

Unlike the other Networks, rather than having specific members, the Transgender Network works through participants involved in varying activities from weekly meetings, to health promoters receiving training. According to Rosa Mayra Rodríguez Lauzurique, Coordinator of the Transgender Network and psychologist at CENESEX, by February 2013, there were approximately 700 participants across the country and approximately 260 in Havana. Moreover, while based in the Center, it also works with groups in four other provinces (Matanzas, Granma, Sancti Spiritus and Santiago de Cuba), as well as working on various training and consciousness-raising initiatives across the island. The Network also assesses each province and the needs of, and support offered to, the transgender community, in order to determine how best to improve their quality of life.

The main group is located in Havana, and is largely made up of transsexuals, who attend weekly or bi-weekly meetings at the Center, where discussions vary from problems with family acceptance, issues with lovers, and general daily struggles. Importantly, the meetings also offer support, from their peers as well as from the Center's staff. The meetings are mainly attended by members of the trans community; but family members, friends, or partners are also often in attendance to offer support or to learn.

The positive effects of the Network on the transgender population are visible at the Center. The main group of approximately twenty transgender people can be seen at the Center for their meetings, or waiting in front of the Center to meet specialists. The group clearly feels comfortable enough to openly discuss their lives in the waiting area, which is populated by other patients or general members of the public, and highly visible to people on the street. They often wait with their partners or friends, and openly discuss a wide range of topics, such as what kind of medication they are on, stage of transformation, dating, clothes and makeup, and the challenges they are facing within their families.

Jurist Network: Red de juristas por derechos sexuales

> "It has been fundamental."
>
> —Manuel Vázquez Seijido, Jurist Network Coordinator, 2013 [Interview]

The Jurist Network is a CENESEX initiative, established at the Center in April 2012, in conjunction with the UNJC. The Center held meetings over three days with law students, as well as various professionals working within the legal profession, to discuss the need for improved legislation regarding sexual diversity rights. As outlined in the Network's 2012 Founding Document ("Documento Base"), there are three main objectives: to question current legislation related to sexual diversity rights; to develop a juridical culture that reflects sexual diversity; and to carry out research initiatives that support the efforts to change legislation regarding sexual diversity rights in Cuba (CENESEX 2012b; CENESEX 2014b). The Network aims to meet monthly to work on the various initiatives and objectives with which it is involved, and also participating with other CENESEX initiatives and programs.

The Jurist Network has been effective in developing legislation and awareness, particularly within the legal profession. It works with the UNJC, which has over 2,000 members across the island, a structure which in effect allows its work to spread efficiently throughout the provinces and legal structures. It is also heavily involved in developing and implementing new courses for law students. For example, the University of Havana's Faculty of Law 2013 course outline and prospectus incorporated themes of gender and legal rights. The courses incorporating gender themes (representing four of the seventy-five courses offered) are available in the provinces of Mayabeque, Las Tunas, and Guantánamo, and are mainly taught by Yamila González Ferrer, a well-known lawyer who works in the development of the island's sexual diversity rights, and one of the primary legal workers on the New Family Code (Goite Pierre 2013; Vázquez Seijido 2013 [Interview]). The Network has continued to work toward increasing awareness and the improvement of legal rights relating to sexual diversity, such as the New Family Code, which aims to establish further legal rights for sexually diverse couples (although it was submitted to the National Assembly in 2012, it is still under debate).

While these Networks have been essential in helping many people, as well as served as a means of researching needs and disseminating information, an ongoing issue is that they are in few provinces, and are almost always focused on the more urban areas. While efforts are being made to expand the Networks to more rural areas, there has been some resistance. This is illustrative of the ongoing problem of the rural/urban divide and the at times sharp contrast in levels of respect for sexual diversity. Nonetheless, the Center continues to include as many areas as possible, and expand the breadth of the Networks in lesser-populated areas.

CENESEX PUBLICATIONS

CENESEX has published a significant amount of work, from *Sexology and Society* (*Sexología y Sociedad*) to books and pamphlets promoting sexual diversity rights through a health-based approach. Many of the publications are funded by international bodies, such as the UN initiatives, but are developed and written by CENESEX specialists.

Sexología y Sociedad

CENESEX's research journal was established in 1994, with funding from the United Nations Family Planning Association (UNFPA). In subsequent years, the material provided in the journal, as well as the frequency of issues, increased rapidly. By the early 2000s, it was published quarterly, with material written by national and international experts in the areas of sexuality and sexual health. It has become one of the most effective means of distributing sexuality-related research within Cuba.

Throughout much of the 1990s, advertisements in the journal focused exclusively on birth control and contraception, as well as on safe and respectful sexual relations. In particular, the use of the contraceptive pill and condoms was heavily promoted (Coll Sánchez 1995; Fiallo 1995). The imagery and vocabulary used for the advertisements was also illustrative of the understanding of sexuality at the time. In terms of vocabulary, the wording for the contraceptive pill advertisements promoted a woman's personal choice and responsibility to protect herself against unwanted pregnancy. This is significant, as it echoes the sentiments regarding abortion as a woman's right. The clear focus throughout was the promotion of women's control over their own bodies and lives.

In campaigns for condom use, the most common words or phrases used included "safe sex," "respect," and "health." The ongoing themes throughout were centered invariably on the importance of engaging in sex in a healthy and respectful way, with an emphasis on one's well-being. It should be noted that the journal was not generally promoting the products of specific companies (with the exception of a few early editions advertising Gynovin as a birth control pill), but rather was promoting the use of the contraceptive method. By the early 2000s, the promotions were largely replaced by many of CENESEX's and MINSAP's campaigns on respect for sexual diversity, and overall healthy sexual relationships.

Analysis of the evolution of the journal is telling, since, while the first edition in 1994 was developed more as a magazine than a journal, it soon changed dramatically. The editions in the early years of publication contained articles about sexual education and sexual health (particularly related to young people), as well as a humor section that had sex-related cartoons, promotions for condom use, and advertisements for birth control pills (Castro Espín 1995; Coll Sánchez 1995; Díaz Noriega and Forbes 1995; Fiallo 1995). Within a few years, the content developed considerably and it evolved into a research journal, publishing national and international studies.

Analysis of the content that was published in the journal between 1994 and 2015 is instructive. When examining all the issues, it becomes clear that the journal has primarily dealt with nine different themes, which are present throughout in the various articles: adolescents; abortions; male sexuality; female sexuality; aging and mature people; community development; sexual violence; those that mention sexual diversity; and those that focus entirely on sexual diversity. Between 1994 and 2015, there were considerable developments in the content, as focus shifted from adolescents and abortion to the question of the normalization of sexual diversity. For example, in 1994, no articles mentioned sexual diversity, while in the following year over 2 percent made note of it. By 2000, 6 percent of articles focused specifically on sexual diversity, and by 2015 over 30 percent dealt with themes of sexual diversity [see Appendix B for complete statistical breakdown].

The content of the articles focused on sexual diversity was comprehensive, including work on specific health-related issues, the history of homophobia, the nature of homosexuality, and social issues suffered by transgender persons. It is noticeable that the work published in the journal was strictly of an academic nature rather than lobbying for, or demanding, improved rights for sexually diverse groups. The journal aimed specifically at education, providing information to readers on various topics, instead of promoting specific political or social demands. Nationally, copies are available free at Cuba's annual book fair, or from the Center itself. CENESEX plans to continue to publish across the island and internationally, increasing the journal's importance and significance.

Books and Pamphlets

CENESEX produces significant numbers of health-related books and pamphlets geared toward different groups or specialists, and covering topics that range from STI prevention, domestic violence, family planning, puberty, communication, gender and sexual diversity, as well as containing instructions on how to hold workshops on a given topic. The material is used for various purposes, including training healthcare professionals (such as medical students, doctors, nurses, and health promoters), helping parents talk to their children, and the provision of education in general. Specific material for the Municipal and Provincial Sexual Education Commissions is also developed, with an emphasis on the prevention of STIs (particularly HIV/AIDS).[8] Notably, the health-based approach is present throughout the literature, and specifically the discrimination-health link.

Similar to *Sexología y Sociedad,* the books and pamphlets are often funded by outside bodies, including the United Nations Development Fund for Women (UNIFEM), the UNFPA, and the Global Fund to Fight AIDS, Tuberculosis and Malaria (GFATM). The significant level of collaboration between various international organizations is illustrative of the quality of the work that is being produced by the specialists at the Center, both in publications and in their professional capacities, as it is their work and studies that are being published with assistance from international foundations. Indeed it is significant that the Center is not being given educational material, but rather is being supported in its efforts to create and distribute its own. Moreover, it demonstrates the importance placed by international bodies on the Center's ongoing work, and their support for its health-based strategy.

Indeed, similar to the earlier work of GNTES, anti-discrimination on the basis of improved health for all has been paramount throughout the literature. For example, a book written by Castro Espín (2003), titled *What Happens To Us During Puberty?* (*¿Qué nos pasa en la pubertad?*), discussed the changes that occur in the body throughout puberty. The book was written for parents (to help facilitate open discussions with their children), and children (since the information is illustrated with colorful cartoons). The section titled "Different?" ("*¿Diferentes?*"), discussed sexual diversity, explaining that during puberty one might develop sexual feelings for the opposite or the same sex, or both. It is explained that this is normal behavior, rather than an illness, and is a part of one's sexual development. As she wrote,

> It is important to know that homosexuality and bisexuality are not illnesses, nor are they immoral. Rather they are expressions of the sexual diversity of human beings. In our culture we have inherited a series of moral values that have established heterosexual relations as being the only "normal" ones. As a result many people unjustly scorn and abuse people who are homosexual or bisexual simply because they are different, and they justify their behavior through reference to beliefs and prejudices that are unsustainable and unacceptable. (Castro Espín 2003, 51)

Each of the published works from the early 2000s includes a section on sexual diversity, where it is discussed as a normal form of sexuality, and condemning homophobia though a health-based approach.

Even pamphlets employ the health-based approach. For example, a pamphlet titled No to Transfobia (*No transfobia*) explains what transphobia is, as well as what a transgender person is (giving definitions for the different categories). The aim of the pamphlet is to increase awareness of transgender people and ultimately to decrease or end transphobia by employing the discrimination-health link. It states that, "Respect for diversity decreases the likelihood of contracting VIH." It also notes that, "The stigma and discrimination to which members of the transgender community are subjected increases their vulnerability to sexually transmitted diseases (STDs) and HIV."

Related publications have historically preceded (and caused) changes in attitudes toward sexual diversity, and can be understood somewhat as a barometer of national attitudes and beliefs. Analysis of the overall published work of the Center since the 1990s clearly indicates a shift toward the promotion of sexual diversity rights. Importantly, as CENESEX is responsible for the materials published, it is unlikely that the work is revised by other ministries, leaving CENESEX almost solely responsible for a dramatic increase in material that highlights the importance of respect for sexual diversity. In addition, it is notable that the most predominant theme throughout is consistently health. The material discusses health as something that all should strive to achieve, while also employing it as a means to normalize sexual diversity.

JORNADA CONTRA LA HOMOFOBIA: CELEBRATIONS FOR THE INTERNATIONAL DAY AGAINST HOMOPHOBIA, MAY 17TH

On May 17, 1990, the World Health Organization removed homosexuality from its list of known mental illnesses. As a result of this change, since 2005, May 17th has been celebrated in many countries, often with parades and speeches, as the International Day Against Homophobia. In Cuba, however, celebrations were, and remain, very different, as the day is used not only to condemn homophobia, but also increasingly to promote sexual health and sexual education, with the aim of promoting overall rights and respect for sexual diversity.

CENESEX organized and led the first celebrations for the International Day Against Homophobia in 2007. While in many countries the day is celebrated with parades, the primary aim of CENESEX's first celebrations was consciousness-raising, with a view to increasing public awareness of issues relating to homophobia and the negative effects of discrimination. It was felt that the means of celebrations employed in other countries (primarily parades) would not be as effective in Cuba, largely due to the country's specific challenges, as a result of its historically rooted *machismo* and homophobia. Thus, the Center sought alternatives to promote the national debate on sexual diversity, employing a model based on education and health. The Center showed a film (Boys Don't Cry), followed by a discussion led by specialists and a public debate on sexual diversity rights. Due to the success of the 2007 celebrations, the Center continued to seek alternative means of promoting the International Day Against Homophobia, increasing the number of events each year (López 2007).

In 2008, in an effort to foster more support for the celebrations throughout the island, the Center requested assistance from MINCULT. The Minister, Abel Prieto, became involved and suggested that, rather than having a celebration or event on a single day, it would be better to make it a week-long event with various activities in order to increase public participation. That year, the celebrations included, among other things, workshops, debates, films, games, lectures, performance art, and the distribution of educational and health-related material (Castro Espín 2013 [Interview]).

Between 2008 and 2015, the celebrations continued to grow in scope, with an increase in participating provinces, and most noticeably in the numbers of people who took part. Notably, there was never a parade as such, but rather demonstrations attended by significant numbers supporting the Day and sexual diversity rights. The demonstrations were, and remain, invariably led by Castro Espín and the CENESEX staff, holding various signs, the Cuban flag, as well as the rainbow-colored flag representing sexual diversity. Amongst the photographs of the demonstration and events, CENESEX staff members, from the head doctor to members of the Youth Network, can consistently be seen, illustrating their commitment to fully participating in these celebrations.[9]

The weeklong celebrations have also gradually increased to fill much of the month of May, with activities occurring daily. The 2012 campaign, for example, lasted from 8 May to 31 May, with a detailed schedule of daily events across much of the island. The schedule for the first day included the inauguration of an exhibition at the Center, followed by a press conference, a panel discussion on the theological inclusion of diversity, and a conference on masculinities. Each day was filled similarly with events ranging from photography and art exhibitions to drag shows, film showings, public debates, theater, lectures, and parties. Along with the increase in activities for the celebrations, the number of national and international specialists involved has also noticeably increased. While in 2007, only CENESEX specialists were involved, by 2014 other Cuban specialists from various ministries and groups also participated in events, such as film crews, poets and writers, as well as members of the Martin Luther King Jr. Memorial Center, and the National Institute of Sport, Physical Education and Recreation (Instituto Cubano de Deporte, Educación Física y la Recreación) (INDER) (for the second year) (*CubaSí* 2013b; *What's on Havana!* 2014, 9). Moreover, the International Association of Gays, Lesbians, Bisexuals, Trans and Intersexuals of Latin America and the Caribbean) (Asociación Internacional de Gays, Lesbianas, Bisexuales, Trans e Intersexuales de América Latina y el Caribe) (ILGA-LAC), as well as specialists from Mexico, Uruguay, Chile, and India were present and involved in panels, debates, and meetings. From 2014, the detailed list of events for Cuba's celebrations for the International Day could also be found in tourist magazines and advertisements (*Prensa Latina* 2014; *What's on Havana!* 2014, 9).

In order to understand the significance of the May 17th celebrations in Cuba, it is also important to consider where and why the celebrations are being held. Many of the celebrations are held in Havana, but other provinces have gradually increased their participation; for example, by 2013, seven of the country's fifteen provinces were participating in the festivities. Indeed it has been an ongoing challenge to incorporate more provinces, particularly the more rural ones, into the celebrations, but this is not just due to problems with sexual diversity, or rooted homophobia. In Cuba, May 17th is also the anniversary of the 1959 Agrarian Reform law, which redistributed large landholdings to the landless. That new legislation was especially important for the Revolution, as it, in essence, fostered support among the rural population, by providing badly needed land to farmers, becoming known and celebrated as the *Día de los campesinos*—or Day of the Farm Workers. It has been annually celebrated, as well as understood as an important part of revolutionary history. Thus, although it highlights the continued struggle to incorporate sexual diversity rights in rural areas, the significance of the celebration of May 17th in support of an International Day Against Homophobia goes beyond support for sexual diversity; it also indicates the importance of the celebration, as considerable numbers choose to share it along with another celebration of great historical importance.

THE "T" OF THE LGBT: NATIONAL COMMISSION FOR THE INTEGRAL CARE OF TRANSSEXUALS

If little is known about the evolution of attention to sexual diversity rights in Cuba, even less is known about the island's transgender community. As there are considerably fewer people than in other groups, they are often omitted from literature, or are represented by a few lines or a short paragraph. In fact *Sexología y Sociedad*'s first article on transgender issues did not appear until 2002 (MacMillan and Yunge Ducaud 2002, 12–14). Yet, for these individuals, their sexual identity can represent a significant health challenge, and affect their wel-lbeing, perhaps more than any other aspect of their lives. For many transgender people, therapy, hormones, support, and sometimes surgery, are needed to achieve a basic level of human dignity (Padrón Durán 2006, 11–19). CENESEX, continuing the work of GNTES, has made a substantial effort to improve the quality of life for the members of this diverse and often ignored group.

The latest published data on transsexuals in Cuba can be found in a book, *Transexuality in Cuba* (*La transexualidad en Cuba*), published by CENESEX in 2008 and written by specialists from various fields, such as law, sociology, and psychology. It explains in detail the transsexual group, including where they live, their approximate numbers, and what their daily lives are like (Castro Espín 2008a, 10). The aim of the work is to bring attention to the daily experiences and struggles of the country's transsexual citizens, humanizing them, and thus promoting their right to healthcare and well-being.

Among those discussed is a transsexual man, referred to by his initials, JR, who had the reproductive organs of a female, but self-identified as a man, which left him feeling "trapped" in a woman's body. He was diagnosed by GNTES specialists in 1972, and was in many ways the catalyst for the FMC's request for MINSAP to support the group's founding of the Multidisciplinary Commission for Attention to Transsexuals in 1979 (Castro Espín 2008b, 23–24; Norandi 2009). Originally from Matanzas Province, in 2008 he was fifty-six years old, was a member of the CDR, Workers' Central Union of Cuba (Central de Trabajadores de Cuba) (CTC), as well as the Civil Defense (Defensa Civil) (DC). In May 1993, he sent a letter to the Minister of Public Health, Julio Tejas Pérez, explaining:

> You cannot know what I suffer day after day because of my situation. I am now 44 years old. I often think that, if I were to have a heart attack and they were to take me to hospital and discovered what sex I am, they would make fun of me and talk about me. . . . That's one of the things that worry me every single day. I think that, if Cuba helps people from other countries, why can't it do the same for me? I am Cuban and my need for an operation is not some passing whim, but rather is based on human need. Only by having this operation will I be able to be a true person. (Castro Espín 2008b, 25)

It was clear in the 1990s that there was an ongoing, and increasing, need for attention to transgender citizens. In particular, legislation that affected their quality of life was extremely rigid, including legislation that made changing one's national identity cards very difficult, which for many often meant that they had to have a photograph, name, and official sex that they did not feel represented them. Specifically Article 31 of Law 51, ratified in 1985 under the Law on Registry of Civil Status (Ley del Registro del Estado Civil), required, among other things, that a person's sex on official documents had to reflect their sexual organs. Following efforts made by CENESEX and MINJUS, a resolution was established in December 1996, according to which changes to a person's photograph or name could be made. As a result, between 1997 and 1998, CENESEX, along with the Ministry of the Interior's "Identification and Registry Department" ("Dirección de Identificación y Registro"), worked on three cases of diagnosed transsexuals, and were able to successfully change the patients' names and photographs, although they were still unable to change their official sex, or other official documents such as birth certificates (Fernández Martínez and González Ferrer 2008, 165–66). In effect, the legislation meant that only those who had received full sexual reassignment surgery were eligible to change their documentation.

In 2004 CENESEX began increasing its work relating to the transgender community, and by extension to transsexual persons. The following year, under Resolución 23 of 9 September, the Center, with support from MINSAP, re-established GNTES' Multidisciplinary Commission as the National Commission for the Integral Care of Transsexuals (Roque Guerra 2009). The Commission was originally going to be named the National Commission for Attention to Gender Disorders (Comisión Nacional de Atención a los Trastornos de Género). However, following significant research, which established transsexuals as constituting a legitimate health and social issue in Cuba and internationally, it was changed to focus specifically on the needs of transsexuals.

The Commission, via CENESEX, sought to assist transgender people, and particularly transsexuals, to achieve the highest quality of life, and improve their overall health and well-being. Transsexuality was understood by the Commission as a mental and physical health issue, and as a result CENESEX sought the introduction of new joint legislation from MINSAP and MINJUS, with the aim of providing necessary care and attention to patients. The Commission worked through various channels, and solicited support from several ministries and organizations. From the initial stages, the PCC was supportive of the Commission's efforts, which were also supported in a December 2005 meeting at the National Assembly by, among others, the Permanent Commission On the Attention to Infancy, Youth and the Equality of Rights of Women (Castro Espín 2008b, 37).

By 2008, the Commission had received ninety-two applications for assistance from various transgender patients. Of the ninety-two patients, twenty-seven were diagnosed as transsexual; two as transvestites; two as effeminate homosexual men; eight left the country (four of these patients had already been diagnosed, while four left before an official diagnosis could be made); while another fifty-seven continued with their diagnostic program. Of those diagnosed, twenty-four were in the "process of changing" (living as the gender with which they idenify) as man to woman transsexuals, and two others as woman to man transsexuals, while one had had the full sexual reassignment surgery and was now considered a woman. Of those diagnosed, thirteen had received their new identity cards from MINJUS, which included new photographs and names. The vast majority of them were living in Havana, while three others were living across the island (Castro Espín 2008b, 26). The Commission has continued to help members of the transgender community, as it continues to engage with both government ministries and the National Assembly to promote rights, and to work on individual cases.

It should also be noted that the efforts made by the Center to care for the needs of the transgender community go beyond the Commission. The Center works through ProNess and its other education strategies with the specific goal of improving the rights for, and decrease discrimination of, the transgender community—including transgender, transsexual, and transvestite groups.

The work of CENESEX undoubtedly developed considerably between 1990 and 2015. The Center's health-based approach was employed in its publications, celebrations, and sexual education programs. Yet, although CENESEX sought to normalize sexual diversity, was the Center successful in its aims? Did it have a significant impact and ultimately the normalization process throughout the island?

NOTES

1. Despite the report being undated and unpublished, the content (including the use of the CENESEX name, as well as specific information regarding HIV/AIDS) suggests that it was written in the early to mid-1990s.

2. Marta María Ramírez is a social communications representative and reporter who has been working for CENESEX for some years. She has worked extensively on the Center's website, participated in public engagements, and has reported on many of the Center's activities.

3. Manuel Vázquez Seijido works as the Head of the Legal Advice at CENESEX. In addition to his legal work at the Center and involvement in legal organizations throughout the country that focus on sexual diversity rights, he is also the coordinator of the CENESEX's Jurist Network.

4. Pedro Pablo Valle Artiz is a renowned doctor, who has worked at CENESEX for several years. He practiced medicine at the Center, as well as participates in many of the Center's academic aspects, such as debates and panels. He was also the coordinator of the Men's Network while this research was being carried out, and worked closely with the Center on the *Jornada Contra la Homofobia.*

5. A psychologist with a Masters in Sexology, Díaz Figueroa worked at CENESEX in various capacities, particularly as the coordinator of the Youth Network while this research was being carried out. He has also published sexual educational material for young people.

6. Ada Caridad Alfonso Rodríguez has served as interim director of CENESEX, as well as sub-director. She has been working at the Center in various capacities as a psychiatrist, and is the coordinator of the Women's Network. She has published extensively on the impact of issues related to sexual diversity, sexual violence, and STIs on mental health and well-being.

7. Rosa Mayra Rodríguez Lauzurique is a psychologist with a Masters in Sexology, and works at CENESEX in many capacities such as sub-director. She is the coordinator of the Transgender Network, and has published widely on themes of sexual education and sexual health, particularly regarding transgender persons.

8. Some examples include, Alfonso Rodríguez et al. 2008a; Alfonso Rodríguez et al. 2008b; Alfonso Rodríguez and González Jiménez 2009; Arrue Hernándes 2005; Artiles de León et al.; Cano López 2009; Castro Espín 2003; Díaz Álvarez 2005; Díaz

Figueroa et al. 2010; Rodríguez Lauzurique 2005; Rodríguez Lauzurique et al. 2009; Quintana Llanio.

9. Examples include, Acosta 2009a; Acosta 2009b; Acosta 2011b; Arreola 2008; *Correo del Orinoco* 2013; *CubaSí* 2013a; *CubaSí* 2013b; Echarry 2009; *elEconomista.es* 2012; Ernesto and de la Osa 2011; *IPS* 2012b; *IPS* 2012c; Menéndez Dávila 2011; *Prensa Latina* 2014; Rowe 2009; Norandi 2009; *What's on Havana!* 2014.

FOUR

Sexual Diversity in Contemporary Cuba, 1990–2015

Between 1990 and 2015, while CENESEX continued to work on specific projects, sectors of Cuban politics and culture were shifting to increasingly reflect the normalization of sexual diversity, as attitudes had changed considerably. This evolutionary process has largely been presented in non-Cuban academia through specific ethnographic studies, mostly conducted and produced in the early and mid-1990s, or, more recently, in literary studies. Throughout these works, authors have attempted to determine why, in the 1990s, attitudes toward sexual diversity shifted considerably.

Stout (2014), for example, proposes that this shift was a result of the Special Period and the political and economic opening throughout the island. She argues that, as a result of the influx of hard currency and the ongoing economic struggle, prostitution, and by extension homosexual sex, increased significantly, contributing to the normalization of sexual diversity. Bejel (2001), by contrast, suggests that the normalization was a result of Cuban nationalist discourse, which evolved to incorporate non-heteronormativity, largely in literature. While both authors, like others, offer insight analysis, they each emphasize a specific component of early change (such as the production of the film *Fresa y chocolate*, or the emergency economic policies and struggles following the collapse of the Soviet Union), rather than incorporating all such factors to form a more comprehensive understanding of the ongoing changes.

It is not the aim of this chapter to speculate on the evolution of attitudes toward sexual diversity from the 1990s onwards, but rather to trace and analyze the process through which they developed. The main events and developments that contributed to the evolution of the normalization in the 1990s, as well as the major areas that have demonstrated change throughout the 2000s will be discussed. In particular, it is clear that healthcare, culture, and politics all played a crucial role in the normalization of sexual diversity.

SEXUAL DIVERSITY IN THE 1990S: HEALTH, CULTURE, AND POLITICS

Health: HIV/AIDS and Homophobia

Cuba's HIV/AIDS experience has been as unique as it has been complicated. Cuban society's prevention and treatment program has often been considered controversial, yet has been highly effective in maintaining Cuba's low prevalence rates—0.1 percent (UNAIDS 2012). Initially, the disease contributed to the evolution of the country's evolving ProNes, while also simultaneously functioning as a means of propelling and increasing levels of homophobia, as HIV/AIDS became understood as a phenomenon affecting homosexual men above all. However, a paradigm shift soon became apparent, and ultimately the disease was used to reduce homophobia, and to increase respect for sexual diversity.

In order to better understand Cuba's HIV/AIDS experience, it is important to first examine how the infection developed on the island, and what the government's response to it was. The first case of HIV/AIDS in North America was diagnosed in 1983, following which the Cuban government immediately founded the National AIDS Commission in an effort to better prepare the country to withstand the infection (Pérez et al. 2004). The Commission was made up of a variety of specialists directed, among other objectives, to design a National Prevention Program for the general population and vulnerable groups, examine and destroy blood reserves, build and introduce a sweeping national epidemiological surveillance system, spearhead scientific research, and establish a national sanatorium system (*Informe de Cuba en virtud de lo establecido en la resolución 60/224 Titulado* 2006; Oxfam International 2008, 5).

Much of the detailed system of prevention and treatment for HIV/AIDS patients in Cuba is based on legislation that was created to minimize epidemics, and to protect society. In other words, the HIV/AIDS epidemic was minimized as a result of legislation that protects the health of the population. For example, one of the most influential laws—Decree-Law 54—was passed on 12 April 1982 (Pérez et al. 2002). The legislation provided the state with the full authority to act in whatever ways it considered necessary to protect the populace from health-related problems. Additional legislation was also created as the threat of HIV/AIDS in Cuba continued to increase over time. The following year, for example, on 13 July 1983 Law 41 was ratified, in which Article 20 referred specifically to diseases that could result in epidemics (Pérez et al. 2004). It stated that:

> The Ministry of Public Health will determine which diseases pose a risk for the community, will adopt diagnostic and preventive measures and will establish methods and procedures for the mandatory treatment, either through ambulatory or hospitalized regimes; and such actions will be conducted by institutions of the National Health System. (Hoffman 2005, 208–9)

In addition, criminal legislation was introduced as a means of protecting the population from health issues. Chapter 5 of Law 62 of the Criminal Code, for example lists punishments for "Crimes Against Public Health." Article 187, Section One, lists the offences and punishments for those who do not follow the guidelines of Cuban legislation; offenders can face significant prison time in addition to large fines (Pérez et al. 2002). It was through these laws that the government carried out its aggressive approach to HIV/AIDS prevention and treatment. This pre-emptive legislative strike proved to be very important for maintaining the island's low prevalence rates, but is also an indication of the considerable efforts made in the early control of the spread of infection. It is also significant that the protection of the country's health rates was viewed as important enough to introduce such sweeping legislation.

Although some media outlets in Cuba at the time suggested that the disease reached the island (with the first official diagnosis in 1985) from a homosexual theatre producer who returned from New York, the more commonly held assertion is that it was a doctor who had returned from a work assignment in Africa (Leiner 1994, 136). In 1986, the HIV/AIDS National Treatment Program was launched, as innovative techniques were employed to contain the growing problem of increasing infection rates. These included the Partner Notification Program, widespread seroepidemiological screening tests, and the development of Cuba's own antiretroviral medications, some of these being highly controversial measures. The most controversial strategy employed by the state was the sanatorium system, in which patients were required (until 1993) to stay in sanatoriums, in order to protect the public from infection, as well as treat the patients (d'Adesky 2003).

The first major center created to assist with HIV/AIDS, the National Center for AIDS Patients, was founded in 1988 in the Pedro Kourí Institute of Tropical Medicine. It was created to study the infection, as well as to provide medical care to patients who required specialized treatment, such as pregnant women. A complementary center was also created in the same year, the National STI/HIV/AIDS Prevention Center (CNPITS-VIH/SIDA). In addition, the two worked closely with CENESEX and the FMC (Fink 2003). In 1988, the ProNes officially integrated information about HIV/AIDS, and in the mid-1990s this expanded to include studies on the optimal teaching methods to provide children and adolescents with necessary information (Álvarez Carril 1995, 38–39).

One of the primary goals of the country's prevention and treatment program was to identify, access, and treat "at risk" groups, such as pregnant women, blood donors, and partners of newly-diagnosed cases. Among them, men having sex with men were identified as a main group of concern, as a result of their comparatively high infection rates. Although homosexual men were considered to be among the most at risk, in terms of infection distribution rates, until the 1990s, fewer homosexual and bisexual men were infected than heterosexual ones. By 1988, for example, approximately 50 percent of those infected with HIV were heterosexual men, approximately 25 percent were women, and another 25 percent were gay or bisexual men (Leiner 1994, 136).

By the 1990s, however, the distribution of HIV/AIDS infection rates changed, and by December 1992, homosexual or bisexual men made up approximately 40 percent of Cuba's infection rates (Castillo et al. 1999). Indeed, the widespread understanding of the infection as a "gay disease" became fully developed in Cuba by the 1990s. As Leiner (1994, 136) asserted, "The perception grows out of pervasive homophobia but is encouraged by exposure to U.S. media reports, which often blame homosexuals for the AIDS epidemic. In the beginning, the Cuban press was not immune to this tendency." Among the issues that compounded this situation was the overwhelming professional emphasis on the improbability of heterosexual people becoming infected. For example, as Álvarez Lajonchere noted in an interview in 1988, the first videos produced on HIV/AIDS implicitly suggested that, if you were not gay, you were probably safe from the infection (Fee 1988, 354). Similarly, a 1989 medical training manual (produced in Spain) that focused on STIs, noted that only between 1 and 5 percent of those infected were heterosexual (Gatell 1989, 183).

The emphasis on homosexuals supposedly perpetuating HIV/AIDS resulted in increased levels of homophobia, and it was still considered for some time as a "gay disease." In many ways, the earlier work of GNTES was overshadowed by the national emphasis on, and fear of, the misunderstood and often misrepresented disease. In terms of medical care, and overall health rates, high levels of homophobia or prejudice made those engaging in homosexual or bisexual sex much less likely to seek and accept medical assistance or follow medical advice for fear of being viewed by either the medical professionals or others as a homosexual. Meanwhile, those engaging in heterosexual sex were unaware of the risks. It soon became clear that the discrimination associated to the disease was creating further health issues, as infection rates and related health problems continued to rise.

As a result of the emphasis on HIV/AIDS in the early 1990s, and the growing understanding of the discrimination-health link, the state sought to implement a sweeping strategy rooted in education and prevention. The need for an increased discussion of sexuality, and thus safe sex, was recognized. In this regard, Leiner (1994, 147) aptly noted, from his study in the late 1980s and early 1990s, that "the Cubans even have the embryo of the organizational structure for this battle in GNTES with its dynamic, knowledgeable leaders." CENESEX thus increased its work on HIV/AIDS throughout the 1990s, incorporating it into its previously-held contention that discrimination was damaging to health.

By the early 2000s, attitudes toward HIV/AIDS had shifted, as the availability of medication, and information regarding the disease, increased. ProNes, as well as CENESEX, dramatically increased their attention to HIV/AIDS prevention, and presented it as a disease that could affect, and infect, both men and women. In other words, the Center highlighted it as an "equal opportunity" disease. The emphasis on the country's preventive health model supported CENESEX's contention that the disease could only be minimized through sexual education and using a health-based approach. The government also began taking more measures to increase sexual education about HIV/AIDS. For example, in an effort to illustrate the reality of the disease, in 2006 a popular soap opera followed the struggles of two men who had difficulties due to contracting HIV (Matos 2006). The result of the disease was a demand for an increase in sexual education, and for specific campaigns (De La Osa 2010, 4).

However, rates continued to increase. By 2005, some 5,422 people were infected. Of them, 80.4 percent were men, of whom 85.7 percent were homosexual or bisexual (Arreola 2006). Three years later, in 2008, the country's numbers increased to approximately 9,000 documented cases, 80 percent of whom were men—and 84 percent of those were homosexual or bisexual. The figures were given at that year's International Day Against Homophobia, noting the need to increase education while decreasing discrimination (*EFE* 2008; *IPS* 2012c).

Importantly, in terms of attention to sexual diversity, the effects were both positive and negative. On the one hand, the disease in effect significantly increased the island's prejudice, albeit for a relatively short period of time, against homosexual men in particular. The fear and misunderstanding of the disease resulted in increased discrimination, and a rejection of sexual diversity, overshadowing and undermining many of GNTES' early efforts. However, the repercussions of the discrimination ultimately resulted in a dramatic increase in the promotion of sexual diversity rights, and ongoing programs. The government, mass organizations, ministries, and specifically CENESEX, increased efforts to employ the health-based approach, and specifically the discrimination-health link to encourage change.

The island's experience with HIV/AIDS served to solidify the discrimination-health link, as it was evident that discrimination against sexual diversity was a considerable threat to individual and national health.

Based upon this understanding, the government increased the role of CENESEX, and the breadth of its work, such as ProNess. In terms of the normalization of sexual diversity, the most significant outcome of Cuba's response to the infection was the understanding that one should confront homophobia in order to confront HIV/AIDS. It became widely understood, following the initial HIV/AIDS crisis, that combating discrimination served to combat health problems.

Culture: Strawberry and Chocolate

In terms of the evolution of attitudes toward sexual diversity, one of the events most commonly cited as a reason for change was the production and showing of the film *Strawberry and Chocolate* (*Fresa y Chocolate*)—with some authors going so far as to refer to historic periods being defined as "before" or "after" *Strawberry and Chocolate* (Rodríguez Boti 2003). It is consistently noted in non-Cuban and Cuban literature on sexual diversity as being one of the most significant milestones in the process (if not the most significant), and is understood to have contributed to the gradual increase in respect for sexual diversity. Yet, like many aspects of this evolutionary process, both the film *per se* and its greater significance have in some ways been misunderstood. Indeed, as Bejel (2001, 156) suggested, the importance of the film goes beyond drawing attention to sexual diversity rights. Instead, he suggests that there are three remarkable things about the film: that it is overtly focused on a variety of social issues, including homosexuality; that it was produced, as well as distributed, in Cuba; and that it was extremely popular, despite touching upon a variety of controversial topics.

Strawberry and Chocolate was released in 1993. The screenplay was written by Senel Paz, a committed revolutionary and the son of a poor couple who were able to dramatically improve their standard of living as a result of changes made throughout the Revolution. Because of those changes, he was able to become a writer, primarily of fiction and screenplays. The film was based on a short story he had written earlier, titled "The Wolf, the Woods and the New Man" ("El lobo, el bosque y el hombre nuevo"), which was published in the late 1980s, and in 1992 was turned into a popular play in Havana. It focused on the friendship between a homosexual man and a straight man with disparate ideologies. The crux of the film was the contention that "Cuban socialism and nationalism must fully integrate the gay (and by extension, the lesbian) members of society" (Bejel 2001, 157).

The film, directed by Tomás Gutiérrez Alea and Juan Carlos Tabío, generated a significant amount of national and international attention. As Bejel (2001, 156) explains, "In addition to winning the prestigious Silver Bear prize in Berlin, *Fresa y Chocolate* was the main attraction at film festivals in Argentina, Brazil, Colombia, Italy, Japan, Mexico and Spain, as well as released in other countries." The film was also later shown in the United States, beginning in New York at a Latin American Film Festival, followed by its subtitled distribution across the country. The film was also extremely successful in Cuba, and was awarded the country's Critics' and People's Choice Awards, along with the Catholic Church's International Catholic Organization for Cinema award for exemplary films (Lumsden 1994, 125).

Although presented as a significant isolated event, or indeed as marking the year that changed attitudes, it is important to consider that, while the film suggested the need to incorporate sexual diversity into the Revolution, it did not function as a singular event that immediately created dramatic change. Instead, it should be understood as simply one component in the ongoing process, and the result of the continuum of change, instead of as a direct cause of it. This can be illustrated by examining an April 1994 interview with Jorge Perugorría, who played the role of Diego, the film's main character, a homosexual man. The article was *Bohemia*'s cover story, as a large photograph of Perugorría was featured on the cover, with the title "I have no interest in causing any scandal: The character of Diego in the film admits that he always exaggerates" ("No me interesa escandalizar: El Diego de *Fresa y chocolate* confiesa que siempre está acelerado") (Terre Morell 1994, 4–6). The article consisted of a three-page spread focusing primarily on his family (wife and children) and future acting aspirations.

Despite playing the role of a homosexual man, and arguably a hero to many marginalized homosexuals, Perugorría consistently made anti-homosexual and discriminatory remarks throughout the article. This is seen most clearly in his answers to two questions that were directed toward issues relating to homosexuality. For example, when asked, "After Diego, what does homosexuality mean to you?," he responded, "It is difficult to give a definition. Everyone knows it. For many it can be a logical, or illogical, attitude toward life." This was overtly discriminatory as it suggests that it is up to one's own opinion, rather than expressing homosexuality as being normal.

In a similar vein, another question asked, "This understanding toward homosexuality, did it come to you after the film?" Perugorría responded that "Look, *machismo* lives alongside us. It's impossible to separate yourself from it. Sometimes, when I was studying gestures, one of my children would see me and I would immediately change it. I didn't want them to see me like that." Moreover, when the interviewer asked how people treat him, he responded by explaining, "No, what happens with my friends is quite different. I live in a *barrio*. My friends live the tragedy of trying to reaffirm that I am not homosexual."

This interview with the star of the film, who played a struggling homosexual character faced with significant prejudice, is indicative of the attitudes toward sexual diversity at the time. Following the film, the island was still clearly struggling with respect for diversity, and issues related to *machismo*. Despite the widespread attention paid to the film, problems of discrimination clearly persisted.

Yet the remarkable and ongoing popularity of the film also suggests that the Cuban audience would at least be receptive to change. It also functioned as a means of reintroducing sexual diversity into the 1990s' national debate in a normative way, rather than focusing on the negative health-related issues that had been prevalent. As a result, instead of being merely a single event that created a dramatic change in Cuban society, its importance can thus be understood as an indication of the changes that had been made leading up to its release, and as a catalyst for future (and increased) changes. The overall significance of the film cannot be ignored, as it remains a critical step in the evolution of Cuba's sexual diversity rights. As Morales Rodríguez (2013) noted, "Twenty years after the story was adapted for the cinema by the same author, and released as *Strawberry and Chocolate*, the story of Diego and David has become the standard reference in the struggle against intolerance."

Politics: Gay Leadership

By the early 1990s, a shift in the attitudes of the revolutionary leadership toward respect for sexual diversity was evident, as public statements began reflecting an increase in attention to related rights, and to anti-discrimination in particular. Possibly the most significant public statement which clearly reflected a dramatic change in attitude, was made by Fidel Castro in a 1992 interview with retired Nicaraguan politician, Tomás Borge. The interview was extensive; it covered topics ranging from Cuban politics to personal experiences, and involved several questions on the topic of sexual diversity and related discrimination in Cuba (and Fidel Castro's personal opinions on it). This interview is almost always noted in work on Cuba's sexual diversity, as scholars have regularly included Fidel Castro's comment, "I am absolutely opposed to all forms of oppression, contempt, scorn, or discrimination with regard to homosexuals." However the significance of the interview goes beyond this singular comment, and is to be found in a large section, including various comments, which expanded on this statement.

As regards to sexual diversity, the two primary questions posed by Tomás Borge were: "The opinion that there is discrimination in Cuba based upon sexual orientation is widely held. What is your view of homosexuality, lesbianism, and free love?" and "Can a homosexual be a dedicated member of the Communist Party?" The first question Fidel Castro began to answer by noting, "You talk of sexual discrimination. I've told you that we have eradicated sexual discrimination" (Castro 1992, 236), and he went on to explain that the Cuban state had worked to end sexual discrimination. He explained that sexual discrimination had been particularly bad toward women, and emphasized the detrimental role of *machismo* in the promotion of equality (including sexual equality), as well as the need to continue improving national attitudes toward discrimination. Specifically in terms of homosexuality, he noted:

> I won't deny to you that, at one point, the whole idea of *machismo* also had an influence on the way in which we saw homosexuality. In my own case—since you are asking for a personal opinion—I don't suffer from that kind of phobia about homosexuals. Really that is not an opinion I have ever held. I have never supported or indeed encouraged any policies against homosexuals. That negative approach to homosexuals was found at a particular period in our history, and is associated with that cultural heritage of *machismo*. I am trying to offer a more human explanation, a scientific explanation of the problem. This situation often turns into tragedy, and is influenced by the opinion of the older generation. Indeed there are some fathers who have homosexual children and can't accept this—it becomes a tragedy for them. You can't help but feel tremendous sorrow upon seeing this, since it turns into a major tragedy for the person involved. (Castro 1992, 236)

While he did not fully address the aspect of the question on "free love," he concluded his answer by explaining simply that he was against discrimination of any kind.

In terms of the second question posed, inquiring if a homosexual could be a member of the Communist Party (which, he had noted in the 1960s that they could not be), he did not explicitly answer. Instead, he noted, "As I am saying, there have been many prejudices around all of this, it's true. It's a reality, and I won't deny it. But there were also other kinds of prejudice, and we instead focused our efforts on overcoming them." While not directly answering the question, he expanded on his earlier statements regarding discrimination, noting that it and prejudice were still prevalent in society, including in the sexual behavior of men and women. He concluded his answer by referring back to the question of "free love," noting that he did not have a problem with such an idea (Castro 1992, 239). This interview is demonstrative of normalization process, and in addition provides a good indication of the ongoing struggles against discrimination. As the leader of the Revolution, and a man considered by many Cubans to be an intellectual, this change in his personal opinion in public from his disparate comments in the 1960s, illustrates the dramatic and considerable evolution of attitudes toward sexual diversity.

In a similar vein, Espín also publicly opposed homophobia in 1992 in a significant public forum. While it was not the first time she had commented in public forums (such as FMC meetings or among colleagues) on issues relating to discrimination and society's rejection of sexual diversity, the comments made in the early 1990s were among the most public (Aguilar Ayerra 2013 [Interview]). For example, she openly corrected the homophobic remarks made by a delegate to the 1992 UJC Congress (Lumsden 1996, 111). Moreover, two years later, in the November 1994 Latin American Congress of Sexology and Sexual Education, when asked if she believed homosexuality should be regarded as a "problem," she stated, "We must still continue struggling in our society to ensure that it should not be so, given that to discriminate against anyone with respect to race, color, ethnicity, religion, sex or sexual orientation, is profoundly unjust and is not acceptable in a society such as ours that has advanced applying genuinely humanistic principles" (Lumsden 1996, 111). This position was particularly significant for lesbians, as, until the mid-1980s, the FMC had at times barred known lesbians from becoming members, and had routinely promoted heterosexuality as the correct family dynamic.

Despite the change in Fidel Castro's public opinion on homosexuality and discrimination, as well as Espín's emphasis on the importance of respect for diversity, few official changes occurred in the 1990s. In terms of legislation, some modifications were made. Most notably, in 1997, Article 303 of the 1987 Penal Code, which classified "taunting with homosexual intention" as a "public disorder," was removed. However other more subtle discriminatory laws remained, such as more severe legal punishments for "crimes of pederasty, when the victim and the adult were of the same sex" (Roque Guerra 2011, 222). Following this shift, it would be about ten years before Cuban politics would incorporate (at times reluctantly) sexual diversity.

SEXUAL DIVERSITY IN THE 2000S

CENESEX increased its work on sexual diversity in 2003–2004, but significant changes did not become apparent throughout the island until 2008. Despite the slow pace of official political change as a result of extensive national debate, as potential changes were carefully discussed and cautiously implemented, other areas have developed considerably, such as published work and increased participation in international and national events on themes of sexual diversity.[1]

Sexual Diversity in Print and Media: Popular-Science, Bohemia, Music and Film

Since the early 2000s, there has been a clear increase in the numbers of works published on sexuality, and specifically on sexual diversity. For example, while earlier popular-science books provided both negative and supportive reports of homosexuality and bisexuality (such as the works of Schnabl [1979] and Brückner [1981], where the authors' competing opinions on sexual diversity were apparent), popular-science works have since evolved to fully incorporate sexual diversity. From books offering relationship advice to those focusing on the sexuality of physically disabled persons, a clear trend has emerged in which sexual diversity is depicted as normal.

The majority of the popular-science books have been directed at young people, and range from those written in a question-answer format to others strictly presenting information on sexuality-related issues. The majority of the work has been published since 2011, and covers topics ranging from teen pregnancy to relationship advice. Among the most prominent writers are Aloyma Ravelo, who has worked extensively with the FMC, and Beatriz Torres Rodríguez, a clinical psychologist, both of whom have based much of their careers on themes relating to gender and sexuality. Between them, they have written a significant amount of the popular-science and advice books on sexuality since 2005.

The most striking difference between the popular-science books of the late 1970s and 1980s, and those published in the 2000s, is the invariable section that discusses diverse sexual orientations as normal. Ravelo's (2005) book *Intimacy: Adolescence and Sexuality* (*Intimidades: Adolescencia y Sexualidad*), for example, has a full chapter dedicated to sexual diversity, called "Homosexuality" ("Homosexualidad"). The chapter specifically discusses lesbianism as well as provides a full analysis of why one must respect sexual diversity. The chapter is written empathetically, not unlike Schnabl's chapter in *Man and Woman in Intimacy*. It notes that, while there had been significant changes since the 1990s in the levels of acceptance, by their very nature prejudices were ongoing, and asserts that society had to make a continued effort to respect diverse sexual orientations. Her other popular books include *About Love, We Speak Frankly* (*Del amor, hablemos francamente)* (1989), *Mysteries of Feminine Sexuality* (*Enigmas de la sexualidad femenina*) (2008), *40 Questions About Sex* (*40 preguntas sobre sexo*) (2009), and *Sex, Love and Eroticism* (*Sexo, amor y erotismo*) (2011). All discuss sexual diversity in a similar way, as she attempts to correct what she calls "myths" about homosexuality, and suggests that a greater respect for diversity is needed. As she explains (2011, 77–80):

> This homophobia, that is, the behavior that is either repelled by, criticises or doesn't accept homosexuality, is responsible for the fact that numerous adolescents and youngsters as well, are uneasy with, reject, or make fun of youths who have another, diverse, sexual orientation. It's a bad lesson that many adults teach to their children from childhood.
>
> What is starting is a real recognition that these people have such sexual preferences. Science has levelled the playing field, but society still doesn't treat us with the proper respect and, although in our country, from the 1990s onwards, you can speak of a greater tolerance . . . but this hasn't been the rapid [change] that we really wanted and need as a society.

In a way that is similar to the work of Ravelo, Torres Rodríguez has contributed to Cuba's published work on sexuality. Her works (2006; 2008) also present sexual diversity as normative behavior, and she asserts that it must be respected. While the work of Ravelo and Torres Rodríguez was possibly the most significant (although it never reached the levels of popularity and scandal that Schnabl and Brückner's work achieved), other authors have written works in a similar vein, such as Miguel Ángel Roca Perara's *Young People With Questions About Being a Couple* (*Los jóvenes preguntan acerca de la pareja*) (2011), which discusses homosexual and bisexual couples.

In addition to the books directed toward young people, work has also continued to be published for other groups, such as books on sexuality for older generations or disabled people. Among them, Rodríguez Boti's (2003) *Sexuality in Later Life* (*La sexualidad en el atardecer de la vida*) is written primarily for older Cubans, which includes a detailed section on sexual orientations. Other authors too have continued this trend, publishing on topics of gender and sexuality (C. Alicia González Hernández and Beatriz Castellanos Simons [2006]; Dulce María Sotolongo Carrington [2011]).

Similarly, there was also a noticeable evolution in the information published in *Bohemia*. While earlier editions devoted a significant amount of their pages to the role of women in the Revolution, in the early 2000s the pages that were once intended to praise women were used primarily as a means of discussing sexuality, specifically of promoting sexual education and sexual health. It is clear from the content and its regularity that sexuality as a concept had, by the early 2000s, become fully incorporated into public discourse and normalized. For example, titles included "The Sexual Vitamin," "Prisoners of Sex," "Sexual Relations," "Speak to your Child about Sex, and "Teenage Pregnancy."[2]

By 2003, while there was a large amount of articles produced on sexuality, their focus had clearly shifted. Rather than emphasizing sexual health and sexual education, they instead focused on how to enjoy one's sexuality. By 2004, these articles appeared at least monthly and increased in quantity and in breadth. The major themes covered were: how to have an equal sexual relationship; the health benefits of regular intercourse; how to have good sex; and male sexual issues. In 2004 there was the first indication of interest in male sexual inadequacies, with several articles on infertility and erectile problems, which for a historically *machista* society, was a noticeable change. In the following years, the range of these sexual topics would continue to increase.

The first comprehensive article about sexual diversity was published in May 2008, titled "Sexual Diversity and Defying Major Challenges" ("Diversidad sexual: desafiando molinos") (Avendaño 2008, 24–28). Following this initial article, there were no further feature articles on sexual diversity, although some focused on aspects of sexual diversity and prejudice, such as "The [HIV/AIDS] Virus Wonders Among Men" ("Entre hombres anda el virus") (Edith and Hormilla 2009, 28–35). Despite its ongoing work on themes of sexuality, *Bohemia* did not publish much work on sexual diversity. This trend suggests the importance of 2008, as the first and only year that a significant article was produced. Despite 2008 being an important year in this regard, the lack of regular publication is also indicative of the continual national debate over sexual diversity and how to address it.

Sexual diversity has also increasingly become present, although to a lesser degree, in music and film. There has been very little published on the topic in music, but we do know that lesbianism has become increasingly apparent in music—in content and artists. Thomas (2006) discussed lesbians as a theme present in music in contemporary Cuba. The song, "Delicadeza," written and performed by Carlos Varela and published in 2003 on his album *Siete,* is probably the first song to have openly and overtly discussed a sexual relationship between two women (Thomas 2006, 133–34). Notably, Varela stated that his intention was not specifically to address sexual diversity rights (and noted that the inspiration for the song came from a painting, *Crema Catalana,* by the Cuban artist known as Cutty). Nonetheless, as Thomas (2006, 133) aptly stated, the song was "a milestone in its own right." Similarly, other singers, such as Gerardo Alfonso have also written several songs about lesbians and their relationships. However, it is important to note that the vast majority of these songs have been written and performed by men (Thomas 2006, 133).

However there have been some examples of females writing and singing about sexual diversity. For example, Yusa is a female singer-songwriter who has written about her own relationships with women. Her most well-known song addressing her romantic experiences with women is probably "Flash," from her 2001 self-titled album, in which she sings about her love for another woman (Thomas 2006, 136).

Themes of sexual diversity have also recently been found in hip-hop. For example, one of the most significant contemporary hip-hop groups, Krudas Cubensi, has actively incorporated women's sexuality and sexual diversity into their music. In 2003 the Cuban hip-hop group, made up of two lesbians, Odaymara Cuesta and Olivia Prendes, released their first album. Their songs address the importance of normalizing sexual diversity (*TeleSur* 2016). According to Prendes, their music is the first time in Cuban hip-hop that that lesbianism and feminism were discussed. The group has also been vocal about the importance of the normalizing process. As Prendes stated in an interview, "music is a very important tool in educating our people and letting them know who we are and what we do. . . . Through music we fight for our rights" (*TeleSur* 2016). While the Cuba hip-hop community is made up mainly of heterosexual men focused on social issues, Krudas Cubensi by contrast continues to produce music that discusses sexual diversity as normative.

Themes of sexual diversity have also been increasingly present in Cuban television. There have been some examples of male homosexual relationships on TV, however the men presented are typically very effeminate and often have HIV/AIDS. A more recent phenomenon has been directed by the FMC and CENESEX's Women's Network, which have been attempting to create more of a space for women's sexual diversity on film. For example, when the Brazilian series *Señora del destino* (which was known to depict sexually diverse relationships) was shown in Cuba, there were obvious points where it had been censored so non-heteronormative scenes were not viewed by the public (Guillard Limonta 2009, 68–69). Following this, CENESEX's Women's Network complained, arguing that, as Guillard Limonta (2009, 69) explained, the censorship "altered the depiction of the realities encountered by a lesbian couple." Despite the complaints, officials in charge of the censorship determined that the information and images were still unsuitable. Nonetheless, it demonstrates the ongoing efforts of CENESEX as well as persisting prejudices throughout the country. Similarly, another program, *Cuando una mujer,* which was supported by the FMC, also demonstrated the ongoing issues with sexual diversity, particularly regarding women in film. While the show depicted lesbianism in a relatively supportive and respectful manner, the word "lesbian" was never used (Guillard Limonta 2009, 69). While sexual diversity in film remains a contentious topic, "nevertheless, it shows that progress is possible" (Guillard Limonta 2009, 69).

Gay Politics

Sexual diversity was not a primary theme in Cuban politics in the early 2000s, and it would be some years before it would become prominent on the national political stage. The first major indication of change came in 2006, as Cuba was among the 100 countries to participate in the "Gay Olympics" in Montreal, Canada. However, significant political policy change would not occur until two years later.

The first major related political shift occurred on 4 June 2008, when Public Health Minister, José Ramón Balaguer (an ex-guerrilla known for his "hard-line" views), signed Resolution 126, which authorized the creation of a center that would provide comprehensive healthcare for transsexuals, including free gender-reassignment surgeries, medication, and therapy (Acosta 2008; Padrón Durán 2006, 11). This was noteworthy because it indicated the first time that the country had offered the surgery since 1988, when the first and only reassignment surgery had taken place. Moreover, it is meaningful that the Minister, who earlier in the Revolution had supported the institutionalized homophobia, was the one responsible for formally approving the decision.

This change followed CENESEX's legal efforts from the late 1990s to achieve improved legal rights for transgender citizens, including the right to change their sex category on legal documentation. It occurred after the Center's other work regarding the transgender community, such as the 2005 Commission for the Integral Care of Transsexual People. Resolution 126 can thus be understood as the political reform that followed the Center's social reform campaigns, as the government steadily increased its attention to sexual diversity in the policy.

Another important moment came in the summer of 2010, when the former president, Fidel Castro, publicly assumed responsibility for much of the homophobia that had been present particularly in the early years of the Revolution. Among the issues noted by him were the UMAP camps, although he blamed much of the discrimination on the cultural influence of *machismo*, as well as on United States threats in the 1960s (*Reuters* 2010). This assumption of responsibility was important, as it encouraged Cubans to re-think what it meant to be a revolutionary. Moreover, it provided an affirmation that changes in attitudes were ongoing. While Fidel Castro did not suggest the need for dramatic policy change, the address did provide a vital step for the respect for sexual diversity, and a criticism of what for decades had been official government policy.

Castro's public address and the 2008 Resolution 126, were thus considered achievements in demonstrating official progressive attitudes dealing with sexual diversity, although it was largely eclipsed in November 2010 by Cuba's role at the United Nations General Assembly's Social, Humanitarian and Cultural Affairs Committee. The Cuban delegates at the Committee voted in favor of an amendment that was proposed by Mali and Morocco, which would replace any reference to "sexual orientation" by the more general expression "discriminatory reason on any basis." In other words, the specific reference to condemning homophobia was replaced by a diluted and more general argument condemning all acts of discrimination. Cuba was one of seventy-nine countries, and the only Latin American country, to vote in favor of the amendment (Acosta 2010a). Thus, while changes had occurred on the island by 2010, in an important international forum, Cuba had clearly taken a step backwards in terms of supporting sexual diversity rights.

Following the vote, CENESEX and SOCUMES were among the first to publicly criticize the government's decision. Alberto Roque Guerra, the former leading physician at CENESEX who also works closely with SOCUMES, stated that, "Failure to specifically mention discrimination on the ground of sexual orientation gives the green light for many states and governments to continue to treat homosexuality as a crime" (Acosta 2010c). CENESEX director, Castro Espín, criticized the decision, while also noting that only two years earlier, on 18 December 2008, Cuba had been among the sixty-six countries to support the United Nation's General Assembly Declaration on Sexual Orientation and Gender Identity, the first statement on sexual diversity and gender identity made by the UN (Castro Espín 2010). This clearly highlights the ongoing national debate throughout the island, and particularly within the political structures. Moreover it demonstrates that change was occurring through a negotiative process, whereby public dissent is not staunchly prohibited in Cuba and that CENESEX was not entirely part of the government structures, nor Castro Espín part of what is often referred to as the "ruling Castro dynasty."

In 2011, the PCC also changed significantly, as the 6th Party Congress officially introduced sexual diversity into its Fundamental Principles, which was later expanded at the 7th Party Congress in 2016. Of particular importance, it stated that discrimination on the basis of race, religion, sexual identity, or sexual orientation would not be tolerated. In addition, it noted that the social and juridical rights of all Cubans, regardless of sexual orientation or gender identity would be upheld (Castro 2012; *Cubadebate* 2011; García López-Trigo 2012; PCC 2016).

These changes were important, as the Party's fundamental principles—the basic concepts on which the Party develops its ideology—changed to officially incorporate a group that it had previously condemned and against which it had previously discriminated. As former Cuban diplomat, Camilo García López-Trigo, noted, "Undoubtedly this is an historic success: for the first time the Communist Party of Cuba has assumed a clear policy against discrimination based upon sexual orientation—and this after decades of silence which have resulted in many homophobic actions, extremely painful for many" (García López-Trigo 2012).

The ongoing shift in Cuba's attitudes toward sexual diversity was evident in November 2012, when the island's first transgender woman was elected at the municipal government level, to become in effect the first known transgender person in the national system of governance. The then fifty-year-old woman, Adela Hernández, was born with male sex organs, though she had identified herself as a woman since she was a child, and had been receiving hormone therapy for the previous three years. She had reportedly suffered degrees of prejudice and discrimination throughout her life, including arrests, and considered her win in the election as an indication of the country's growing respect for sexual diversity (Rodríguez 2012; Progreso Semanal 2012).

Of particular importance to the evolutionary process and development of rights was the development of the New Family Code and its submission to the National Assembly in October 2012, outlining amendments to include gender and sexual diversity under the law. It is unclear when the idea for a New Family Code (that is, an amended version of the 1975 Code) developed. According to Castro Espín, it had been an ongoing project of the FMC since the early 1990s, as FMC members sought advice and suggestions from various specialists regarding possible improvements needed as a result of the ongoing socio-cultural and economic shifts facing families (Castro Espín 2007, 3). Indeed, as with its predecessor, the development of the New Family Code was an evolutionary process based on national debate and reflecting contemporary needs.

Between 2005 and 2007, the need for an amended Code became more apparent, and official discussion began, the aim being to develop a Code that reflected the reality of Cuban families, which were no longer necessarily the heteronormative ones presented in the 1975 version. The primary organizations that were responsible for developing the new Code were the FMC and the UNJC, working in conjunction with CENESEX, which largely provided data and suggestions. Like the first version, the FMC sought various opinions about what to include and what to exclude. Debates and meetings were held with representatives from almost every major group or organization, including the Church, FEU, and UJC. Similarly to the initial Family Code, it was the aim of the organizers to include as many participants as possible, in order to create the most fair and acceptable Code. The idea being, that if people were involved in the dicisions and debates, they would later be more likely to accept and respect it. As a result, several versions were written over the years, with the earlier versions including a section whereby same-sex couples could adopt, as well as enter into a lawful marriage. The negative popular feedback regarding the adoption rights of same-sex couples, as well as the specific reference to "marriage," prompted the adoption amendment to be dropped, and the change of the term "marriage" to that of "civil union" (Vásquez Sejido 2013 [Interview]; Ramírez 2013 [Interview]).

Throughout the negotiation of the new Code, two central themes remained evident. The first was the inclusion of the concept of gender, rather than sex, in order to to reflect the contemporary needs of men and women. While one's "sex" refers specifically to sexual organs, "gender" is a social construct that generally reflects a male or female identity; a man could have male reproductive organs but his gender could be female. Gender as a concept was believed to be an important addition to the Code in order for it be more inclusive of sexual diversity. The second theme was to reform the rights of non-heteronormative citizens, to provide recognition of the rights of sexually diverse persons and their families. These included civil unions, and the right for lesbian women to have access to the country's *in vitro* treatments, among others. Overall, the aim of the New Family Code was to make the idea of family more inclusive. As Acosta aptly noted, "The reformed Family Code would stipulate that the family has the responsibility and duty to accept and care for all of its members, regardless of their gender identity or sexual orientation" (Acosta 2008).

The New Family Code was presented to the National Assembly in October 2012 by UNJC Secretary, Yamila González Ferrer, one of the Code's primary activists. However, the process for the amendments to be agreed upon and ratified in the Assembly is extensive and largely based on a series of drawn-out debates and approvals. The process involves discussion in various debates and negotiations over specific conditions, with amendments being suggested and discussed by members of the National Assembly. Following this, it is presented to the entire Assembly, largely as a summary of the Code, followed by further debates and ultimately a vote. Moreover, if the vote is carried, there is another complex process to turn it into legislation. If the vote fails, a newer version does not need to be resubmitted, as the Assembly will keep the initial proposal and reassess it at a later date.

In 2017, the Code was still being considered and open to debate, but beyond that little was known regarding the stage it was at in discussions. The amendments to its predecessor remained an ongoing topic, as CENESEX and other organizations such as the UNJC and FMC continued their efforts to persuade the National Assembly to incorporate diverse family structures into laws. CENESEX in particular has continued to press for a change to the island's Family Code, as well as to support all legislation that reflect sexual diversity rights. As noted by Castro Espín, if the rights of sexual diverse Cubans are not ratified, then they are in essence left unprotected by the law (Sierra 2008).

Meanwhile, with the significant advances in incorporating sexual diversity into the political agenda, the 2013 Labor Code (otherwise known as Ley 116/2013) prompted considerable debate (*Antiproyecto de Ley Código de Trabajo* 2013). The Labor Code was originally instituted in 1985, with various amendments made over the following decades. The "new" Code was produced in 2013, and published for the public a full six months after it had been fully analyzed, debated, and finally agreed upon by the National Assembly. Since it pertained to many of the new changes in Cuba's economy, it received a significant amount of international attention. What the newspaper and reports did not pick up on, however, was that, in addition to the anticipated changes regarding employment legislation, the Code also propelled further debate over the question of sexual diversity, as many felt that it was in some ways discriminatory.

The majority of the criticisms focused on Article Two, which stated that

> The fundamental principles that govern the right to work are a) every woman or man who is fit to work, without distinction of race, skin color, sex, religion, political opinion, national or social origin, and anything else that is detrimental to human dignity, has the right to obtain employment with which they can contribute to society's goals, satisfy their needs and those of their family, and serve the demands of the economy and of their choice, as much in the state sector as in the non-state sector. (*Antiproyecto de Ley Código de Trabajo* 2013)

While some considered it a victory, if only a minimal one, for the island's sexual diversity rights, others felt it was a discriminatory piece of legislation. The most common complaint was that this section in particular did not make reference to sexual orientation or gender identity, and rather placed them under the umbrella of "anything else that is detrimental to human dignity." The lack of specific regard to non-heteronormative citizens, it was argued, also went directly against the PCC's fundamental principles regarding discrimination. Moreover, it has also been argued that it focused specifically on men and women, omitting and thus discriminating against transgender citizens. Various bloggers, activists, and members of CENESEX's Networks, among others, have since continued to criticize the Labor Code's lack of specific protection for members of diverse sexual orientations and identities.[3] While the Code remains an area of contention, it is illustrative of the ongoing political issues in terms of accepting and representing sexual diversity. Although significant changes have occurred in politics across the island, problems persist.

Contemporary Medical Training

In Cuba the field of medicine, and specifically medical training, has steadily increased its emphasis on the importance of sexuality and sexual diversity in its curriculum. As a result of the persistence of CENESEX, more courses have been offered throughout medical universities on the needs of sexually diverse patients, and sexual health overall has become a priority in recent years, as the medical field has increasingly considered sexuality to be an important indicator of health and well-being.

Unlike the evolution of treatment of patients with HIV/AIDS in Cuba, the incorporation of sexuality, and particularly sexual diversity, into medical training is still very new, and there is little information on it, apart from a clear increase in ProNess' efforts within the field. That said, a good example of change in medical training is the 2013 launch of SEXSALUD. As Noides Manuel Bell Fernández, a Youth Network leader in the province of Santiago de Cuba and sixth-year medical student (at the time) noted, "it is called SEXSALUD, a fusion of the words sexuality and health, because we want to treat sexuality from a perspective based upon health" (Puentes Valladares 2013a). Based in the University of Medical Sciences of Santiago de Cuba, it is a program whereby medical students have access to online chatrooms that cover various topics including sexual violence, adolescent sexuality, sexual rights, sexual diversity, sexual health, and STIs (primarily HIV/AIDS). Within the chatrooms are specialists (such as CENESEX personnel and various medical professionals) who offer information and advice to the medical students (CENESEX 2013; InfoMed 2013).

While the program lasts only one week, with two hours in the morning and two hours in the afternoon available in two computer labs for students to participate, it is a clear indication of the means with which the government, and MINSAP in particular, are aiming to increase medical training on issues of sexuality. The government, undoubtedly, sought to meet the demands of the medical field. Moreover, it also indicates CENESEX's ongoing emphasis on training younger generations, including medical professionals, who will be able to better address the needs of different sexual groups, while reducing discrimination.

Another clear indication of the incorporation of sexuality into the medical field is the changing curriculum at the Latin American School of Medicine (Escuela Latinoamericana de Medicina) (ELAM). The original aim of the school was to provide medical training to people from marginalized and underserved regions across the world (Castro 1999). MINSAP, via CENESEX, has been working to incorporate sexual diversity into the medical training. One of the first examples of this was a 2012 debate during the celebrations for the International Day Against Homophobia, in which CENESEX specialists participated, along with medical students, on topics of sexual diversity and particularly homosexuality. While some students were very uncomfortable with the idea of learning about sexuality, others noted that it was an important part of medical training. Since the initial debate, ProNess and MINSAP have continued to increase their emphasis on sexuality in medical training at the school.

The fact that MINSAP is investing in the promotion of international attention to sexual diversity through medicine is significant. This example, as well as SEXSALUD and the other areas of ProNess, illustrate that medical training is being used to decrease prejudice through the discrimination-health link, and ultimately increase respect for sexual diversity. The underlying message is clear, that in Cuba health and healthcare can be used as a vehicle to create and develop change.

ONGOING PROBLEMS: DISCRIMINATION, PREJUDICE, AND VIOLENCE

There have undoubtedly been major changes in the normalization of sexual diversity in Cuba since 1990. Yet, while it is important to note the evolution, it is equally important to understand the ongoing areas of difficulty and challenges, such as enduring levels of discrimination and prejudice.

The ongoing problems with the normalization of sexual diversity are not unique to Cuba, although they are illustrative of the continuing evolutionary process on the island. Among the most significant problems is persistent discrimination and prejudice. This is evident from the clear differences in visibility of sexually diverse persons throughout the country. Like most countries, Cuba's capital and other major cities have a higher number of sexually diverse citizens, largely because of the anonymity that living amongst a larger population provides. In Havana, for example, seeing gay (male or female) couples is not uncommon, and this has visibly increased in the last ten years, while in other more rural provinces, it would be very uncommon to see two men holding hands. The areas where sexual diversity is more noticeable reflect a higher level of acceptance and respect, whereas in other areas many same-sex couples feel uncomfortable demonstrating their sexual orientation publicly (Roque Guerra 2013b; Roque Guerra 2009).

The lack of visibility of sexually diverse couples and related problems of discrimination are also apparent in national cultural productions, such as those on TV and the radio. As previously mentioned, lesbians in particular are very rarely discussed or shown, while male homosexuals are often presented as very effeminate and infected with HIV/AIDS (Acosta 2009b; Matos 2006). There has also been criticism of having sexually diverse people presented in the media, as some citizens believe that this perpetuates bad or dangerous sexual behavior (Arreola 2006). It is clear from both the visibility of sexually diverse people as well as responses to them, that discrimination is ongoing on the island, chiefly in less populated areas where *machismo* is often more intense.

Violence against sexually diverse persons has not been a focus of any normalization campaign or sexual education literature. By contrast, violence against women, children, and adolescents has been widely researched and has been, for many years, central to sexual education as well as a theme that the FMC has been actively involved in. In order to bring awareness to sexual violence, there are frequently art shows, booklets, studies, and all sexual education literature invariably includes sections or chapters that addressed the importance of preventing violence, including sexual violence against women, children, and adolescents (Rivero Pino 2014; Chávez Negrín 2011; Centro Cultural Pablo de la Torriente Brau 2012; Díaz Tenorio et al. 2011). The central theme to preventing and protecting against violence, and similar to that of normalizing sexual diversity rights, has been that of a health-based approach—including the protection of mental, physical, and psychological health. As one pamphlet condemning violence against women noted, "violence increases the risk of contracting STIs and HIV/AIDS" ("Tu condición de mujer" [n.d.]). While these campaigns, research, and publications are extensive, they focus exclusively on women, children, and adolescents. There is little, if any, discussion of violence against sexually diverse persons, and they continue to promote mostly heteronormative values.

Indeed, while many measures have been enacted to protect some groups or communities against violence, sexually diverse citizens have, for the most part, not been among them. A specific issue has been that of hate crimes in particular. Although the topic is slowly gaining momentum in some of the island's research circles, there have been very little data collected on hate crimes related to sexual diversity. Research on the topic mainly began in the early 2000s, with a study aimed at measuring levels of psychological and physical violence suffered by homosexual couples. The study, conducted at the Centro Provincial de Educación para la Salud de Santiago de Cuba, and carried out by psychologist Pedro Oscar Telles, discovered that, of those studied, approximately 94 percent had experienced psychological violence, while 48 percent were reportedly victims of physical violence (Acosta 2009b). Other studies have also suggested that, of the sexually diverse groups, transgender persons suffer the most psychological and physical abuse (Chávez Negrín 2011, 206–7).

Levels of homicide as a result of sexual diversity are also indicative of ongoing prejudices. González Pagés (2014b), for example, noted that in 2013 there were over forty reported homicides across the island as a result of hate crimes against sexually diverse persons (primarily homosexual men and transgender persons). Among those killed were significant public and cultural figures, including dancer and choreographer Alfredo Velázquez, economist Eduardo Pérez de Corcho, and director and stage designer Tony Díaz (González Pagés 2014a). While the exact number of homicides each year in Cuba is unknown, it is clear that it is a relatively low number compared to its Latin American neighbors and it is thus likely that those killed via hate crimes represented a significant percentage of the overall rates.

Despite the problems with violence, it is important to consider that the category of "hate crime" in Cuba is relatively new, and demonstrates the growing attention to the specific needs and problems associated with sexual diversity. It is unlikely that, before 2000, crimes against homosexual men, or transgender persons, would have received the significant attention they have received in recent years. While the figures highlight a problem of violence toward these groups, equally the attention to this level of violence demonstrates the overall evolution of attitudes. In other words, despite it being a clear problem, the fact that the problem is not being ignored suggests in itself a dramatic change.

While the Cuban media, as well as the international media, focus more on the positive aspects of the evolution of attention to sexual diversity rights, it is important to consider the necessary areas for improvement. In particular, respect (rather than tolerance or acceptance) for sexual diversity could still be improved considerably. Moreover, violence against sexually diverse persons must be discussed in ProNess, as well as be addressed in the media. In the same vein, the media and cultural outlets must continue to increase the presence of sexual diversity. Indeed, despite significant advancements in the area, challenges remain, as the island, and CENESEX in particular, continue to work toward improving sexual diversity rights and attention to diversity.

Between 1990 and 2015, there were significant shifts in attitudes toward sexual diversity. What becomes evident from examining the normalization process is that the health-based approach, and especially the discrimination-health link, was essential. Yet it remains unclear why health was such a focal point for this process, and why a health-based approach was employed. We are left wondering why this normalization process happened this unique way. What was it that made health more important to the Cuban government and population than the traditions of the historically rooted *machismo*? How did health become so important to revolutionary Cuba? Do Cubans interpret health and healthcare differently?

NOTES

1. For example, Bonilla 2007; Castro Espín 2004; Collazo 2010; *EFE* 2013; González Delgado 2013; *Juventudrebelde.cu* 2007; Leyva and de Armas 2010; Menéndez Dávila and Omar Parada 2010; Nova 2010.
2. These articles can be found, for example, in *Bohemia* 2001a, 69; *Bohemia* 2001b, 69; *Bohemia* 2001c, 69; *Bohemia* 2001d, 69; *Bohemia* 2001e, 69.
3. Among them, Díaz 2014; Paquito 2013; Roque Guerra 2013a.

FIVE

Cuban Healthcare

What Is Different About Health in Cuba?

Revolutionary Cuba is not unique in its belief that health and healthcare are critical to development, but the country has become known internationally for its attention to health, which has been a priority since the beginning of the Revolution. For example, in July 2014 the Director General of the WHO, Margaret Chan, visited Cuba, where she noted the state's commitment to the provision of healthcare: "Cuba is the only country I have seen which has a healthcare system closely linked to closed-loop research and development. This is the right direction to be moving in, because human health cannot improve without innovation." She also stated, "I keep a special place in my heart for Cuba and recognize the efforts of the Cuban government to establish health as an essential pillar of development" (*Granma International* 2014). However, despite international acclaim and studies on the evolution of healthcare, few, if any, observers have offered suggestions about why it has developed. Good health rates have undoubtedly been an aim of the Revolution, but thus far academics have not really offered explanations on the reasons for this. In other words, we know *how* the healthcare system works and has evolved, but not *why* it works and has evolved that way.

WHY DO GOVERNMENTS AND INDIVIDUALS CARE ABOUT HEALTH?

Health has always been of paramount importance to societies and individuals. For some countries, one of their greatest accomplishments is considered to be their healthcare systems, such as the United Kingdom and its National Health System. By contrast, other countries' governments have hit a crisis point, such as in the United States, where the government even briefly stopped functioning as a result of arguments over a national health scheme. Indeed the virtual implosion of the U.S. government in 2013 due to "Obamacare" is telling. Moreover, many global regions are characterized by their poor health statistics. Sub-Sahara Africa and Haiti, for example, are areas that have become synonymous with HIV/AIDS and low life-expectancy rates.

Analysis of the literature on health, healthcare and Global Health suggests four main reasons why health, and by extension healthcare, is valued: specialists note that it is an important aspect of productivity; it is an indication of a country's level of development; it is a human right; and it is vital to individual (and by extension, national) well-being.

There is a clear understanding that, in terms of productivity (of a country or an individual), a healthy worker is a productive worker (Gauri 2003). While authors have suggested that various aspects of health contribute to higher levels of productivity, including nutrition, levels of disease, and fertility rates, the central concept in all the arguments is that, in order to be more productive, an individual or society must be healthy. In a similar vein is the understanding that epidemics are expensive, and should thus be avoided so as to maintain production rates. The financial costs of epidemics are felt across governments, private companies and societies, as every level is affected. Undoubtedly, this cannot be viewed as a blanket understanding across all histories and cultures, as the relationship between health and productivity is complex. Nevertheless, it does provide a valuable contribution to the overall understanding of why health and healthcare are valued by both societies and individuals.

A second reason why health is valued is that it is considered an important indicator of a country's individual level of socio-economic development, with a particular emphasis on the role of the state (or in most cases the strength of the state). Health is understood as a significant indicator of a country's profile, suggesting the level of the state's stability, infrastructure, GDP, gender equality, and quality of education. Health is used as a barometer of a country's development, and is believed to be the measurable result of a complex relationship between other development factors, such as education and gender equality. It is also viewed as the result of a state's ability to provide the necessary factors that contribute to improved health rates. Thus health is understood as important because it can be used as an overarching measurable indicator of development (Harman 2012).

The third reason why health matters is that it is considered by the United Nations, amongst others, as a basic human right. This concept relates to Adam Smith and his contention regarding the importance of "the ability to appear in public without shame" (Smith 1776, 469–71). The right to health is fundamentally important for one's self-respect (Rawls

1971, 60–65). Health as a human right, then, is important as it provides (in theory) a basic equality for all persons, the aim being that everyone is entitled to a basic level of respect. Health is a vital component of that basic respect, so that a person can exist with the highest possible level of dignity.

A final reason that health is cared about beyond the "live-longer" argument, which supports the idea of health as a human right, is that it is a significant contributor to one's sense of well-being. While the definition of well-being has been contested and developed in different disciplines, it can best be understood as a level of happiness, or contentment with conditions, vital to the way in which an individual, or a community, wishes to live. As Wiseman and Brasher (2008, 358) explain, "Community well-being is the combination of social, economic, environmental, cultural, and political conditions identified by individuals and their communities as essential for them to flourish and fulfill their potential."

Well-being was introduced into discussions of international bodies in the 1950s and 1960s, since, while it was previously believed that a population's level of happiness would increase alongside its economic development, data suggested that this was a misconception. Since then, measuring a country's or a region's well-being has become increasingly important and complex, and there has been growing attention paid to it, as greater numbers of specialists and international bodies increase their interest and problematize previously held assertions. Health is clearly a significant contributor to individual and community well-being, and, importantly, it is measurable.

Although all four of these can arguably be seen as separate reasons to explain why health matters, it is important to understand that they are all interconnected and interdependent. Production, development, rights, and well-being are aspects of a global socio-economic framework. Production may be principally the reason why health was historically important, but social development ideas also shifted the emphasis to rights and well-being. These four reasons work both as separate entities and as complementary ones, as health and healthcare have continued to reflect both moral and economic concerns. However it is important to consider that for revolutionary Cuba, it was a somewhat different experience.

EVOLUTION OF THE CUBAN HEALTHCARE SYSTEM

The Revolution's healthcare system developed from 1959 to provide universal healthcare to the population at no cost to patients, while dramatically increasing the numbers of medical professionals, and has (for several decades) boasted some of the best health data in the world, and with very little help from international bodies. Its model has worked outside the confines of traditional healthcare systems, generating international interest and research.

Some authors, particularly from the United States, have criticized the system, suggesting that it significantly reduces personal agency, and does not support human rights (Powell 2004, 92). Moreover, as Huish (2013, 33) has argued, a common perspective among critics is the belief that an economically weak country could have nothing to teach the larger, more affluent countries. Yet the majority of academic research lauds the country and system for their efforts in developing and maintaining a strong healthcare system and health rates. The healthcare system has been studied at length, with writers largely focusing on the system's evolution, or key components of its fundamental make-up, and notable health rates. Even former World Bank president James Wolfensohn noted, "Cuba has done a great job on education and health care. . . . They have done a good job, and it does not embarrass me to admit it" (Kirk and Erisman 2009, 46).

Revolutionary Healthcare in Cuba: General Principles

Cuba's revolutionary healthcare system can best be described as following a community-based participatory model. The emphasis began by stressing curative measures, but soon evolved to incorporate the importance of prevention. Yet throughout the development of the healthcare system, the implementation of community medicine as the vehicle for health improvements has been consistent. Health and healthcare were viewed by the population, as well as the state, as being a national responsibility—requiring the active participation of all members of society. From the outset, the understanding of health in Cuba went well beyond the view of being simply a lack of illness, and rather promoted well-being based on bio-psycho-social determinants.

In terms of understanding the island's complex healthcare system and view of health, it is instructive to understand the three complementary pillars on which it was built and developed. The first is that healthcare is a human right. The revolutionary system has emphasized this from 1959, and it is even outlined in the 1976 socialist Constitution of the Republic of Cuba, which noted that

> Everyone has the right to the care and protection of their health. The State guarantees this right: By offering free hospital and medical services. . . . By offering dental treatment; By developing plans for sanitary efforts, health education, periodic medical exams, general vaccination, and other preventive medical means. In these plans and activities the entire population participates through the social and mass organizations. (Asamblea de Poder Popular 1995, 23–24)

This view has been central to the system's development, and the state's commitment to its provision. The second pillar is that healthcare should be free and accessible. A clear understanding, and latter expectation, of the provision of healthcare is that this should be provided at no cost to patients, and should be accessible regardless of geography. This has been a consistent principle concerning the provision of healthcare throughout the Revolution.

Finally, the third pillar is that health and healthcare are the responsibility of the state and general population, and must emphasize prevention and participation (Rojas Ochoa 2003). Ernesto "Che" Guevara, himself a doctor suffering from considerable health problems, discussed at length this view of healthcare as well. He stated, for example, that, "One day medicine will have to become a science that serves to prevent diseases, or orient the entire public toward their medical obligations, and that only has to intervene in cases of extreme urgency to perform some surgical operation or to deal with something uncharacteristic of that new society we are creating" (Guevara 1997, 127). By this he was referring to the belief that health is not an individual phenomenon, but rather based on society and social determinants. This understanding has been translated into an emphasis on community health and participation, particularly in regards to prevention, as being critical to developing and maintaining a healthy population. This principle is rooted in the view that health is the product of competing bio-psycho-social dynamics, and must thus be promoted and treated through various channels.

In essence, the three pillars suggest that health is complex, and healthcare must be strategic. In other words, that it must focus on the particular problems of a given area, and continue to develop multi-faceted and multi-sectoral means of improving it, with the ultimate aim of improving health rates. Moreover this insistence on the provision of free, accessible healthcare for all is illustrative of the importance placed by the Revolution on participation and prevention.

Pre-Revolutionary Cuba

While much of the literature presents a positive view of healthcare in Cuba after 1959, it is important to consider that, before the Revolution, the island also had one of the most advanced healthcare services in the Americas. The island had a long history of healthcare options and medical training, from 1726 when medicine was first taught in Cuba, and 1728, when the University of Havana was founded, with a Faculty of Medicine (Morales Suárez et al. 2008, 5). The faculty maintained a reputation for excellence in medical training, following much of the syllabi of American medical schools, and in addition required students to take the U.S. medical board exams.

Despite the high quality of medical training and care (available at the island's only medical faculty, at the University of Havana), it was almost completely unavailable to the vast majority of the country, geographically and financially, as it was almost exclusively private and centered in urban areas (primarily Havana and Santiago), and largely serviced the wealthy (Hirschfeld 2007, 204–5). Thus, while the services offered were comparable to developed countries, they were very poorly distributed, even among the few who could afford them. MacDonald (1993, 25) describes pre-revolutionary medical services well as an "urban business enterprise." He continued to state (1993, 101) that "medical services represented yet another business to which the poorest sectors of the population had no access, and if they did, the services were of the worst quality." The health-related disparities were particularly bad in the 1950s, as Cuba had one of the highest doctor-to-patient ratios in the Americas (approximately 1,078 patients per doctor in 1958), although fully 65 percent of medics and 62 percent of hospital beds were in Havana. This figure is more staggering when one considers that half the population lived outside the city, and only one rural hospital (with ten beds) existed throughout the country (Kirk and Erisman 2009, 27; Navarro 1972, 413). Overall, the health of the population was very poor—particularly for those who lived far from the capital.

The country's health and healthcare were central to Fidel Castro's 1953 defense speech, which became known as "History Will Absolve Me." Used to defend the rebels' actions in attacking the Moncada Barracks as being justified by the Cuban Constitution, it cited various areas of Cuban governance that were in a desperate shape. Among the issues were the country's health problems and distribution of medical care. He stated that

> Ninety per cent of the children in the countryside are consumed by parasites which filter through their bare feet from the ground they walk on. Society is moved to compassion when it hears of the kidnapping or murder of one child, but it is indifferent to the mass murder of so many thousands of children who die every year from lack of facilities, agonizing with pain. (Editorial de Ciencias Sociales 1975)

In the speech he repeatedly made reference to the need for improved healthcare, and noted that it would be among the principal revolutionary changes. It was thus evident from the outset that health would be a focus of the Revolution.

Stage One: Transition, 1959–1969

In 1959 the delivery of healthcare began to change dramatically across the island, resulting in improved health statistics. Fidel Castro appointed Julio Martínez Paéz as Minister of Health. He had been a revolutionary throughout the struggle against Batista, and the government set out to improve the delivery of healthcare. A new medical system and a new form of doctor based on empathy and *humanismo* began to emerge almost immediately. It was believed that a new system required a new type of doctor, who was dedicated to providing healthcare at no cost to patients, rather than providing it for profit.

The provision of doctors and infrastructure became priorities, resulting in the re-opening of the University of Havana in 1959 after it had been closed by the Batista government three years earlier. The medical school resumed courses, despite having only 23 of its 161 teachers remaining on staff. The others had either emigrated or refused to teach (Morales Suárez et al. 2008, 5). Moreover, there was a mass exodus of nearly half of the country's doctors and surgeons in the following years, as only 3,000 of the country's 6,000 remained on the island. The courses at the university also changed to fit Cuban health needs. For example, the government discovered that the Department of Pediatrics had never researched, and thus was not instructing on, the three highest causes of child mortality in Cuba (parasitic infestation, usually intestinal; gross malnutrition, which in Cuba's case this typically meant starvation; and diarrhea caused by enteric infections, leading to death by dehydration) (Kirk and Erisman 2009, 37). While physicians were being trained, doctors from other countries volunteered to practice temporarily in Cuba, and medical students in their last two years of training were used also.

Training also shifted in the early years of the Revolution toward community medicine, rather than individualized care. For example, the 1960 Law 723 outlined the necessity of training health workers in social welfare issues (MacDonald 1993, 136). Moreover, since the 1960s, medical graduates were required to pledge their commitment to practicing in the public health system, and to provide care to anyone who required it, at no cost to patients. This suggests an early and clear emphasis on the importance of community medicine, as various psycho-bio-social factors were being considered.

The increase in human resources also contributed to the establishment and expansion of medical care in rural areas. Act 723, established in 1960, of the Revolutionary government, created rural medical services based on recently graduated medical students who were required to work in rural areas (designated by the government) for one year (originally six months), a period that was later increased to two years (Pérez 2008, 42). This was also known as the Rural Social Medical Service (RSMS), which employed increasing numbers of recently graduated medical students in rural and underserved areas (Huish 2013, 37).

The initial role of the rural doctors was to treat communicable diseases and major health issues such as tuberculosis, leprosy, venereal diseases, pregnancy, children's acute diarrhea and malnutrition. The emphasis on treating the symptoms of patients gradually changed, as the medical personnel became fixtures, and often leaders, of communities. An undated mimeographed MINSAP report titled "Rural Medical Service Information Pamphlet," presumably from the early 1960s (because it discusses the work of the initial waves of rural doctors), noted that:

> The doctors lived in people's huts, where they also saw patients. . . . At first, their role was purely to care for the sick, given the huge numbers of people who came to see them daily. With time, as doctor-patients relationship developed and as doctors became more integrated into the communities, their social and educational role came into its own. (Morales Suárez et al. 2008, 6)

The report concluded that "the doctor has become an important figure in these rural communities, establishing a relationship never seen before with local people" (Morales Suárez et al. 2008, 6).

In addition to the RSMS, one of the most significant changes in terms of health provision in the early years of the Revolution was the development of polyclinics. Originally established in 1962, the polyclinics were critical in developing comprehensive public healthcare. Staffed by a doctor, nurse, OB/GYN, pediatrician and social worker, they were used to provide public healthcare, while participating fully in local health initiatives (such as campaigns, and specific drives focusing on vector control) (Whiteford and Branch 2008, 20). They also provided disposal instruction and health condition inspections within the community. Moreover, they worked with other participating community-based organizations and groups, such as the FMC, CDRs, National Service to Eradicate Malaria, and social workers.

During the first decade of the Revolution, the objective was primarily to control and treat disease. Yet the role of the new medical personnel and infrastructure was clearly in the process of increasingly shifting focus to primary care through a participative community medicine strategy. Through 1959–1969, the aim of healthcare shifted—although maintaining a community medicine strategy—from treatment to primary care.

This could partially explain the FMC's insistence on free and safe abortions in the 1960s, as the numbers of doctors increased, as did the geographic areas they covered. By this stage, health and healthcare had already become a priority of the Revolution, and particularly women's health as it related strongly to population health. Indeed, it could more easily be argued by the FMC that safe abortions were reasonable, among the various others reasons discussed in earlier chapters, if free and accessible healthcare was already being emphasized by the state.

Stage Two: Structure Public Health, 1970–1989

In the 1970s, the transition stage that sought to develop the previous medical system into a sweeping public healthcare system began to focus primarily on structuring the new medical system. In other words, while until 1970 the government worked to implement a new public system, the second stage of development was the specific structuring of the system. Once the understanding of a public system was established, the nuts and bolts of that system also had to be developed. Between 1970 and 1989, the government developed a comprehensive structure for the public healthcare system, providing primary, secondary and tertiary care.

As previously noted, one of the early and significant aspects for the revolutionary healthcare system was the establishment of municipal polyclinics. In 1974 an extensive analysis of the polyclinics was carried out, with a view to identifying problems and proposing solutions (Gardner 1981, 16–17). A main problem was that they had failed in some ways to integrate medical specializations, as each team of specialists worked separately instead of working as one complementary team. An additional problem that was identified was that they were not working principally within a community medicine framework, and were instead prioritizing curative-based medical practices over preventive care (*MEDICC Review* 2013, 3).

As a result of these critiques, the polyclinics increased their role within the community, as well as their lists of primary care services. These included the provision of clinical services, environmental services, community health services, and related social services to a specifically defined area of population. The clinics' directors also worked with various other health officials, to review health initiatives and maintain communication channels (for example regarding new policies, programs or results) (Danielson 1985, 52). In essence, they can be understood as a means for MINSAP to have a significant and direct role in the community. These polyclinics became a critical component of the primary care model, and continued to develop over time, as needs and strategies progressed.

By 1975, significant progress and a dramatic increase in attention to healthcare were evident, and were reflected in health statistics. For example, between 1958 and 1975, the National Health budget increased from $22,000,000 to $400,000,000; the number of blood banks from one to twenty-two; medical schools from one to four; nursing schools from one to thirty-four; and doctors from 6,000 (although approximately 3,000 left) to 10,000. Moreover, the number of annual diagnosed cases of polio decreased from 300 to zero, malaria from 3,000 to zero, diphtheria from 600 to zero, and gastroenteritis from 4,000 to 761. Furthermore, infant mortality decreased from sixty per 1,000 live births to 28.9, while life expectancy increased from fifty-five years to seventy (MacDonald 1993, 29).

In an effort to continue to develop the healthcare system, in 1976 a five-year comprehensive plan was introduced to continue integrating medicine and medical professionals into the community, with an emphasis on preventive rather than curative care. The aim was to increase community medicine, with a focus on primary healthcare. There were, however, ongoing problems regarding the accessibility of medical professionals, particularly outside the polyclinics.

In the 1980s, the community medicine strategy was expanded to incorporate the innovative Family Doctor Program. Launched in 1984, the program sought to place a doctor and nurse team in every neighborhood—one team serving approximately 150 families. They worked in their *consultorio* in the morning, and spent the afternoon visiting patients in their homes in order to better understand the lives (and lifestyles) of the community members. This allowed the doctors to analyze possible health risk factors (diet, exercise, smoking, sanitation), while becoming familiar with the members of the neighborhood. The goal was to "break down barriers between doctors and patients, by making the doctors members of the communities they served," as well as increase the accessibility to medical professionals and care (Hirschfeld 2007, 214).

The program served to enhance community participation in health, making it a collaborative responsibility of individuals, communities, and medical professionals. Although the Family Doctor Program worked outside the polyclinics, it is important to consider that they functioned to complement the services offered there. The program worked well, and by 1986 "each Cuban medical school was offering a postgraduate degree to qualify as a family doctor" (Kirk and Erisman 2009, 43). The Program fitted well into the island's three-tier medical strategy: the Family Doctor Program provided primary care, the polyclinics secondary, and hospitals focused almost exclusively on tertiary care.

Stage Three: Emphasis on Community Medicine, 1990–2006

By the 1990s, significant success had been achieved in the provision of, and access to, healthcare. The number of polyclinics had increased from zero (in 1958) to 391, and the number of hospitals from 97 (in 1958) to 264 (MacDonald 1993, 63). However, the country faced major challenges following the collapse of the Soviet Union, which spilled over into its Public Health system. In terms of health and healthcare, what happened over the next ten years was revealing of the island's commitment to healthcare provision.

As a result of the considerable decrease in calorific intake, between 1992 and 1993, Cuban males lost on average thirty pounds; between 1992 and 2001, 60,000 people suffered from optical neuropathy, due mainly to vitamin deficiency; and between 1990 and 1993 the rate of low birth weight in newborns increased from 7.6 percent to 9 percent (Huish 2013, 41). Moreover, materials and medication were scarce, as pharmacies had very little to offer patients, medical personnel often had to wash and recycle gloves and syringes, and hospital patients were often required to bring their own food and bedding. An additional problem was the decision of medical staff to leave their positions either for economic reasons (often seeking employment in the tourist sector) or for lack of motivation, as they had to practice medicine with few or no resources.

Yet, while economic challenges, and as a result health problems were ongoing and at times increasing, the government maintained its focus on the importance of public health. As Fidel Castro stated in 1992 at a Santa Clara University graduation ceremony for medical personnel, "Even if we stop building hospitals and health care centers until 1997, Cuba will retain its privileged position as having by far the most successful public health system of any other third world country" (MacDonald 1993, 15).

In particular, two complementary strategies were implemented in order to maintain good health rates and universal healthcare: the continued training of medical professionals to increase their numbers, and an emphasis on community medicine. As one specialist explained,

> In the mid-1990s, the MINSAP began a new period of transformations in the sector, its goal to define main strategic lines and programs that would lead to system consolidation and modernization, including new methods and styles of work. Since that time, increasing health expenditures have limited spending in other public sectors. (Iñiguez 2013, 45)

In terms of the numbers of medical professionals, it is clear that these continued to increase throughout the period. Indeed, it is important to consider that, during the economic crisis, the government did not close a single hospital or university, and even increased enrollments on medical training courses. For example, in the 1990s, nearly 38,000 doctors graduated, approximately four times the number that graduated two decades earlier (Morales Suárez et al. 2008, 7). By 1999, there were 66,000 practicing doctors, and 2,200 medical school graduates entering the system each year, and, with one doctor for every 169 people, Cuba had the best doctor-to-patient ratio in the world (Huish 2013, 43). This suggests an ongoing belief in the value of trained medical professionals, and of access to them by the general population.

The second, and complementary, strategy that was implemented was an emphasis on community medicine. While it had been a significant element of earlier decades, as a result of the economic tension and absence of resources, it became the focal point of the public health system (Neusy and Plasdottir 2008, 20–24). The belief was that an increase in community medicine would translate into an increase in prevention of disease, and thus enable the struggling healthcare system to sustain and even improve health rates. One of the primary ways that community medicine was emphasized was through concentrated medical training, focusing on the prevention of disease. As had happened in previous years, medical training shifted to promote this new view. A MINSAP commission, for example, outlined 286 common health problems, which graduates would be required to identify and treat at the primary care level. Basic health problems became central to teaching, as prevention was again emphasized over curative measures (Morales Suárez et al. 2008, 6). Doctors were, in essence, being trained to participate in a new community-based medical system, in which clinical medicine and population healthcare were integrated.

Other areas of the healthcare system also shifted to participate in community medicine, as MINSAP continued to assess health problems and "outline strategies for sectoral recovery centered on improving service quality, efficiency and effectiveness and on maintaining equity" (Iñiguez 2013, 45).

The gradual emphasis on prevention of health issues through a community medicine approach played a significant role in the health-based approach employed for the normalization of sexual diversity. While the discrimination-health link was established in the 1960s, and continued to be used by GNTES throughout the 1970s and 1980s, it was not until the HIV/AIDS crisis of the late 1980s and early 1990s that this link was solidified and understood by the government and populace as important for maintaining and improving national health rates. Preventing HIV/AIDS was clearly more important at the time than curing it, and it was evident from earlier experiences that discrimination was detrimental to this aim. Beyond HIV/AIDS, the understanding of prevention over curative means would also apply to all health concerns, as prevention was viewed as less expensive and more effective. This mentality in Cuba of the tremendous importance placed on prevention between Stage Two and Stage Three would have been largely responsible for the widespread support and implementation of the health-based approach employed to normalize sexual diversity. The discrimination-health link, and the subsequent national and individual health benefits, worked because prevention was an integral part of the Cuban healthcare ethos, and the particular community-medicine model practiced. It was thus important to inculcate in the medical personnel, as well as the population that discrimination was detrimental to health—a strategy that would continue to be employed.

Stage Four: Expanding Community Medicine, 2006–2015

While writers such as Whiteford and Branch (2008), Bravo (1998), and Danielson (1985) have posited that the healthcare system has followed three stages of development, similar to those outlined in this chapter, more recent data suggests that there is a fourth. While it could still be considered as a continuation of the third stage's emphasis on community medicine and accessibility, an argument could be made that it should be categorized as a different and new stage altogether.

The development stage from 1990 to 2006 emphasized community development, as well as accessibility of medical services. Since then, however, it is important to consider that the understanding and provision of this medicine in the community has broadened considerably, and has fully incorporated an understanding of well-being. To explain, the same strategies have continued to be implemented (such as increased technologies, polyclinics, medical training), although other aspects of citizens' well-being have been considered. This includes an increased emphasis on other areas of health, such as nutrition, social policy, communication, and psychiatry, as well as a greater emphasis on other areas of studies such as sociology and psychology.

In a 2006 interview with *Temas*, Francisco Rojas Ochoa, one of Cuba's most well-known and respected doctors, articulated a hypothesis of what future changes could occur in the healthcare system, "I would hope for—I don't know if this is what will happen or not—something closely tied to training a physician who pays more attention to the social dynamics of health and disease. More health promotion . . . greater attention to social problems that affect human health" (Iñiguez 2013, 50). Several significant changes have occurred in recent years in the delivery of healthcare in Cuba. Among these are medical professionals learning about the psychological and mental health issues associated with sexual diversity due to prejudice; the effects of nutrition on mental health; and the various contributing factors to one's well-being. In other words, healthcare seems to embrace more fully the view that health is not simply the absence of illness or disease.

Moreover, in 2010, the government instituted the "reorganization, consolidation and regionalization of health services." The central goal of this was to re-emphasize the importance of community medicine and the prevention of health-related issues on all fronts, while decreasing reliance on tertiary care, and thus high-tech treatments. This example again supports the contention that the concept of community medicine has been gradually expanded since 2006. The government continues to reorganize healthcare based on the needs of the population, resulting in a greater understanding of health, and how to achieve it. In addition to the discrimination-health link, a broader understanding of health has been essential to the normalization process, as it highlighted throughout the medical profession that sexual diversity is an important part of well-being. In other words, that being content with one's sexuality has an impact on one's well-being. Moreover, additional aspects related to anti-discrimination, such as domestic violence and hate crimes, became health issues as well as criminal issues.

Today Cuba's healthcare rates and system are considered by many scholars and specialists as comparable, if not better, than those of many developed countries. For example, 99.4 percent of Cubans have regular access to healthcare, and Cuba's doctor-to-patient ratio is one to 170, which is better than the United States' one to 188, and better than any G8 country (Huish 2013, 45). Furthermore, as a 2009 study by Kirk and Erisman (2009, 45) discovered, "Cuba allocated 23 percent of its central government expenditure to health and 10 percent to education, while the

United States allocated 22 percent to health, and 2 percent to education." Moreover, Cuba spends approximately $251 annually per person on healthcare, while the United States spends $5,711 annually per person, and Canada spends $2,989 (Pérez 2008, 5). These disparate data are suggestive of the Cuban government's and populace's commitment to their healthcare system, and its effective strategy on prevention and provision.

WHY THE CUBAN SYSTEM EVOLVED

Significant attention in academia has been placed on how the Cuban system evolved and how it works, as authors have outlined stages and provided supporting data. Yet, no study has offered an understanding of *why* health and healthcare were, and remain, a focus of the Revolution. Why did the government emphasize free and accessible healthcare? Why did doctors work in underserved areas? Why did the number of doctors increase throughout the Special Period? And, beyond that, what was the role of health as a priority for the Revolution in the *imaginario* of the political system?

As noted earlier, there are four principal reasons why health is generally and globally viewed as important (productivity, indication of development, human rights, and well-being). Yet it is important to consider that for revolutionary Cuba, it was a somewhat different experience.

The evolution of the provision of healthcare in Cuba suggests five main complementary reasons as to *why* health and healthcare were emphasized strongly by the Revolution. These include the personal commitment of Fidel Castro, morality, production, equality, and *humanismo*. These reasons should be understood not as competing, but rather, like the reasons suggested within the Global Health framework, as complementary. They have been corresponding elements behind the evolution of Cuba's healthcare system, and offer greater insight into *why* the system evolved as it did.

The first of these was the personal commitment of Fidel Castro to the universal provision of healthcare, at no cost to patients. Although it can be argued that an individual could not be responsible for a country's commitment to the provision of healthcare over a span of several decades, in the case of revolutionary Cuba, the former president's personal commitment was significant.

It is clear from his speeches that he maintained a profound personal belief in the importance of healthcare. As previously noted, it was among the changes he wished to institute in his 1953 defense speech, and remained a theme of his speeches from the beginning of the Revolution.[1] For example, as he stated in a speech in 1978, "There are even some developed countries that need doctors because they don't have doctors to send to some [marginalized] areas. And in the situation of those countries exploited by the colonial powers, the situation is truly tragic. Tragic!" (Castro 1978). His commitment to the provision of healthcare at no cost to patients was undoubtedly a main reason for Cuba's overall commitment to it as well. His role must be understood as a driving force behind the island's development of healthcare.

The second reason that can be drawn from the evolution of the island's emphasis on health and healthcare was a fundamental belief in morality, and the moral imperative to provide healthcare to the population. This moral belief began at the beginning of the Revolution, and continued to develop throughout. In pre-revolutionary Cuba, health and healthcare were freedoms extended only to those who could afford them. For instance, while there was a comparatively large number of doctors at that time, most worked within a strictly monitored private framework. In addition, there was a clear division between the provision of medical care in urban and rural settings, with the latter being at a serious disadvantage. For many, healthcare existed but was inaccessible, and, as was the case with so many other difficult conditions, was the result of ongoing structural violence. For this reason, in the early years of the Revolution, the provision of universal, accessible healthcare made available at no charge by the state can largely be attributed to an emphasis on basic morality.

This revolutionary view of morality was rooted in the belief in human dignity, that is, the idea that every human being deserved a basic and universal level of dignity. Many poor Cubans had not been afforded their dignity, due to economic conditions; thus it became the moral imperative of the Revolution to provide its citizens with a basic level of quality of life and dignity. The provision of healthcare was understood as a means of providing this basic level, so that Cubans could live and work without the shame caused by illness. For many, who had been living in very difficult conditions and dying young, this was a considerable moral coup.

It thus began as the view of the government, that universal health was a moral imperative and fundamental human right, one that should be made available to all Cubans, regardless of their social standing or location. While it began with the leadership (among them, this was an evident belief of Guevara, who wrote extensively about morality and health, as well as Fidel Castro, who often discussed health in a moral framework), it also influenced the views and actions of doctors and graduate students. Healthcare in fact as a moral imperative was a clear reason behind the initial push for improved health rates.

This also occurred during the period when many Cubans felt, and eventually affirmed, that they were creating a socialist society. It was understood by the government and much of the population that the Revolution was working within a socialist framework, as Fidel Castro professed in April, 1961. This also strengthened the government position on curative medicine, as a result of the sweeping medical issues that were prominent in the early 1960s, mainly among the poor and marginalized. Morality was undoubtedly the primary reason for the Revolution's focus on health in the beginning. Yet as curative measures improved the health profile of the general public, and universal healthcare was increasing across the island, a shift in the reasoning also occurred.

The third reason why the Revolution focused extensively on health and the provision of healthcare was the need for greater productivity. This is not meant in the clinical way that the word may imply, but instead reflected an understanding that the Revolution could not advance if the population was not healthy. In other words, health was a priority because it would allow the Revolution to consolidate and expand; an unhealthy population could not contribute to, or participate in, this process. Healthcare was thus a logical step in the advancement of the revolutionary aims, which ultimately sought to promote equality.

The importance of productivity is particularly evident when considering Cuba's experience in reproductive health, and especially abortion rights. This strategy is evident throughout the 1970s, as the various institutions of the Revolution, including the mass organizations and ministries, worked to dramatically improve conditions across the island, and industrialize the economy as much as possible. Health was directly linked to these developments, and thus productivity. The healthcare system developed at this time to incorporate community medicine and emphasize prevention, in an effort to develop and maintain a healthy population, able to fully participate in all aspects of the development of the Revolution.

In addition, the Revolution needed to develop the capacity to focus on specific aspects of healthcare delivery, such as the need for improved infrastructure and trained specialists in order to change attitudes regarding the country's health (such as the importance of community participation in prevention). It took several years to establish the means and capacity to educate people on health. The emphasis on a strong national healthcare strategy was thus linked to the production needs of the country—mainly a population that could participate in and advance the Revolution.

The fourth reason for the prominence of health within revolutionary Cuba was from the start, and still is, equality, which is not surprising given the socialist nature of the revolutionary process. In other words, the inequality of being ill resulted in a healthcare system rooted in equality—health was used as a means of creating basic equality.

Although it could be argued that it was simply a result of, or possibly the continuation of, the morality that has been instilled in the early years of the Revolution, it is the contention of this study that the government's insistence on accessible healthcare goes well beyond that. The belief in the importance of equality was thus one of the primary reasons for attention to, and development of, healthcare.

The understanding of the essential nature of equality in health evolved, from practical equality (such as basic goods and services) in the initial stages of the Revolution to a view of health as being a means of maintaining a basic level of equality within the Revolution's population (such as during periods of economic challenges and advancement, including the Special Period, and more recent national economic opportunities). In other words, health developed from the provision of a service to the maintenance of a basic level of equality throughout the revolutionary system. During the various challenges that Cuba has faced, both national and international, health and healthcare have been constant throughout. It was one of the elements that was distributed equally among the different socio-economic strata—the Minister of Education, for example, was to receive treatment comparable to that of a rice farmer.

Health equality is also an important means of Cuba competing in international standings, as the island's expertise in healthcare has often been used to promote the country as equal or comparable to industrial ones, at least in this regard. Health has been used as a means of maintaining Cuba's identity as an equal to other countries, despite its considerably fewer financial resources, and of fostering relationships (economic and diplomatic) with other countries. The emphasis on health and healthcare is thus used to maintain the island's international standing as being equal to some of the wealthiest and most powerful nations.

The importance placed on equality in health also extends to well-being, particularly since the early 2000s. Returning to the earlier view at the beginning of the Revolution regarding morality and human dignity, in contemporary Cuba well-being and one's right to live with dignity have re-emerged as important facets of healthcare. It is the view of MINSAP that healthcare must provide an environment conducive to one's well-being. While basic services were once provided, the system has evolved to provide a variety of services that support health, as well as to promote the importance of the role of the community in the provision and maintenance of well-being.

Probably the clearest example of this approach, and one directly pertinent to the subject of this study, is the way in which health is used to promote respect for sexual diversity. Indeed, while in the 1960s doctors were providing immunizations, today they are running awareness-building training, and working to fully incorporate sexual diversity into the healthcare system in an effort to improve health rates and decrease levels of discrimination. Respect for sexual diversity has clearly been understood as being important to well-being and one's individual self-dignity, and as a result has been gradually (albeit at times reluctantly) incorporated into the healthcare field.

Therefore, the idea of the equal distribution of healthcare as a main factor in the evolution of healthcare in Cuba since the 1970s is indeed a complex one. It cannot be reduced to the maintenance of revolutionary influence, nor should it be understood romantically as a simple act of empathy, or an act based on moral imperatives. Instead, it is a combination of such factors, as well as of other competing factors, including the personal emphasis placed on health by revolutionary leaders.

Equality is a theme present within the Revolution, and is presented in various ways and areas, and in this case it has been used to promote health within the revolutionary framework. It is malleable and significant, and will continue to be employed within the field of healthcare. The importance of equality in health can be seen and felt across the island, as no matter what economic changes occur, healthcare promotes a basic equality between all citizens.

The final reason that health and healthcare occupy such an elevated position within the Revolution is the core belief in solidarity, and in particular, an understanding of *humanismo*. For revolutionary Cuba, *humanismo*—the belief in the importance of humanity, the value of human life, and by extension the responsibility to both respect and protect it—forms the cornerstone of its medical practices and ethos.

The term *humanismo* has been used in Cuba in various senses throughout the Revolution's history. It is another means of explaining human "force" or "willpower" (Castro 1964), yet it invariably refers to the basic belief in the human condition's need for a good quality of life. While the power of the term is somewhat lost in translation, the word is distinguished by what revolutionary Cubans understand as the essence of being "human"—solidarity.

However, the belief in *humanismo* as a reason for Cuba's sustained emphasis on healthcare has not been articulated in any of the literature on the subject. Nor is this concept necessarily qualitative or quantitative, and so it does not lend itself to sustained rigorous analysis. Wider academic research has yet to offer any reasons why the revolutionary system has focused so intently on health and healthcare. However, while being aware of the difficulties of trying to define something as nebulous as *humanismo*, this study offers this explanation as the result of extensive research and experience, and as an attempt to put a name to Cuba's healthcare system, and the many who participate within it.

The Cuban healthcare system has clearly developed separately, and in many ways differently, from others. In particular, the Cuban system has developed in a way that is significantly different from that of other developing countries. This in itself is not necessarily new information, as researchers have frequently noted the impressive difference in health rates between Cuba and other developing countries. That said, analysis of the system and its development, particularly following the 2006 shift to the expansion of community medicine and an emphasis on well-being, is instructive. It supports the contention that Cuba has a good healthcare system, while also suggesting new dimensions to our understanding of the system. Indeed, analysis of the Cuban healthcare illustrates the commitment and participation of both the state and the general population, as they engaged in the negotiative process of the evolution of their healthcare and how it was provided. Cuban problems were fixed with Cuban means.

It is also important to consider that the Cuban system has worked almost entirely outside the influence of neoliberal governing bodies that have consistently directed Global Health governance since the 1960s. When the island was in the midst of the economic crisis of the 1990s, the problems were not dealt with by seeking World Bank or International Monetary Fund (IMF) loans that ultimately resulted elsewhere in the privatization of health and in the increase of market forces. While there was some funding provided from the UN as well as some NGOs, this funding was largely controlled by the Cuban specialists who were free to determine how to best spend it. The healthcare system in Cuba was able to develop almost entirely independently.

While Global Health understands the reasons for the importance of health and healthcare in terms of production, development, human rights and well-being, the Cuban system promotes a different reasoning. In Cuba, the emphasis on and belief in productivity, morality, equality, and *humanismo,* in addition to the personal commitment of Fidel Castro, has resulted in health and healthcare being viewed differently than elsewhere. The reasons differed in much the same way as the development strategy of Cuban healthcare, which was primarily based on community medicine rather than financial gains.

This suggests that for Cuba, solidarity was and remains more important than strictly financial incentives. The country's belief in the importance of health and healthcare has been rooted in human dignity above all.

NOTE

1. Including, among others, Castro 1963a; 1963b; 1964; 1969.

Conclusion

(R)evolution

The evolution of attitudes toward sexual diversity in Cuba is not unique, as many countries have normalized sexual diversity to varying degrees, particularly since 1990 when homosexuality was removed from the WHO's list of mental illnesses. What *is* unique is the way in which attitudes changed in Cuba, as until now there has been almost no explanation about *why* this considerable change occurred. The reasons behind the island's significant changes in attitudes toward sexual diversity have never been clearly evaluated, let alone described with contemporary evidence to accurately represent these changes.

The process of the normalization of sexual diversity in revolutionary Cuba is as interesting as it is complex. Scholars have recognized the island's particular version of homophobia in the early years of the Revolution, and have attempted to trace its progress. The volume of work that was produced in the 1990s on homosexuality in Cuba is illustrative of the wide interest in this Caribbean country's experience with sexual diversity. Most of that work was largely completed in the early 1990s, while the extensive media reports began around 2008—yet there has been no indication of what happened in the almost twenty years in between. What is clear, however, is that the attitudes toward sexual diversity in contemporary Cuba are very different from those from the 1960s and 1970s. Indeed, as we have seen, the island was once notoriously homophobic, but has in recent years been lauded for its attention to sexual diversity rights, with no explanation of how this change occurred. We thus began this book by asking how attitudes toward sexual diversity evolved in Cuba.

In order to illuminate this question, this study has therefore examined the country's revolutionary history of anti-homosexual attitudes, and also explored the role of the FMC and the early development of sexual education and sexual health. It has demonstrated that the FMC was critical in this regard, since attitudes toward sexual diversity began to change as a result of the organization's early efforts to promote reproductive health and sexual education. Importantly, the FMC established the discrimination-health link through its work to legalize safe abortions. This link would prove to be of paramount importance in normalizing sexuality and later, sexual diversity. In effect, sexuality and the importance of sexual health were incorporated into the national debate and normalized in the early years of the Revolution as a result of the FMC's efforts, particularly through GNTES.

The evolution of CENESEX, the missing component in earlier studies, also proved to be crucial to the normalization process. The fact that the Center has been working under the auspices of MINSAP implied clearly that sexuality was important to national health. CENESEX thus increasingly developed sexual education, and later specifically began emphasizing sexual diversity in 2004, as by then the topic had become incorporated into national debate, and it was clear that further information and attention were needed.

Finally, this study has explored the importance of health and healthcare in Cuba, and in particular traced the development of the healthcare system, and thereby answered the question of why health and healthcare were, and remain, so important in revolutionary Cuba. Between the analysis of the island's homophobia, of the FMC's work in sexual education and sexual health, of the role of CENESEX, and of the island's emphasis on healthcare, some clearer answers to the *why* and *how* have emerged.

Until now, it was widely believed that the changes in attitudes could largely be attributed to the 1993 release of *Fresa y Chocolate*, which functioned as a catalyst for change. It was believed that, as a result of the film, the Cuban government and population gradually began accepting homosexuality, and incorporating related anti-discrimination into official policy. From around 2008, it was also believed that Castro Espín, as the daughter of Raúl Castro and the niece of Fidel Castro, had the power and influence to institute considerable change. It has been further posited that, through CENESEX, she pushed sexual diversity rights forward into the national agenda. These have been commonly held views to explain why attitudes have changed. Although this understanding is not entirely incorrect, as both the film and the Center, led by Castro Espín, have been powerful influences on the development of the normalization of sexual diversity, the interpretation is far from accurate. What has become evident is that this evolution has been far more complex. Change was not the result of a film, an organization, or the work of an individual; it was a far more involved process, spanning the length of the Revolution.

The significance of establishing a more comprehensive understanding of the normalization process goes far beyond reinterpreting previously held assertions, or challenging the work of other scholars. Instead, it is important to consider the question of why the strategy itself is unique. It is not uncommon for countries, even those with a *machista* reputation, to promote respect for sexual diversity; Uruguay and Spain for example have legalized marriage for same-sex couples. So why is the Cuban case important? What is it that makes it special?

We can now conclude that changes occurred in Cuba as a result of a health-based approach, which emphasized the discrimination-health link. Unlike in other countries or strategies, the normalization of sexual diversity in Cuba was not achieved on the basis of human rights, but rather employed a strategy rooted in health. Although rights for sexually diverse groups were among the aims, the health-based strategy implemented first by the FMC and GNTES, followed by CENESEX and ultimately the government, focused on health to normalize sexual diversity. The central theme of this strategy was the fundamental understanding that discrimination was detrimental to individual and national health. Notably, the Cuban health-based approach is the first time that this strategy has been employed.

The preceding chapters have demonstrated that the discrimination-health link began early in the Revolution. The FMC, following the success of legalized abortions based on the discrimination-health link, argued that discriminating against the sexuality of lesbians was detrimental to their health, as they would be less likely to seek medical attention, or follow medical advice. Although it was initially employed to advance sexual and reproductive health, it soon evolved to incorporate sexuality, specifically sexual diversity.

By the late 1970s and early 1980s, this strategy was also highlighted throughout much of the literature that was produced on sexuality, and began to incorporate sexual diversity. Schnabl's *Man and Woman in Intimacy* had an entire chapter dedicated to sexual diversity, and the principal argument used there was that of health. Similarly, although his books that were published in Cuba suggested that homosexuality was deviant behavior, Brückner's underlying message throughout was that safe and respectful sexual relationships were important to one's health and well-being.

The spread of HIV/AIDS in the early and mid-1990s also reinforced the discrimination-health link, as it was believed that those who were infected, particularly men, would be less likely to seek medical treatment, or follow medical advice, because of prejudice against their perceived sexual orientation. This view was not unlike the position concerning sexual health for women that was promoted in the 1960s. While the infection initially affected homosexual men particularly negatively, including increased levels of homophobia, in effect it functioned as a catalyst to incorporate education about sexual diversity more fully into the medical field.

Throughout the Revolution, sexual education increasingly became a model and a device to promote healthcare, reflecting the belief that safe and positive sexual relationships, of whatever gender, were important markers of both individual and societal health rates. In particular, it was viewed as the vehicle through which individual and national sexual health would be achieved. It is clear from the evolution of the FMC's role, as seen in the establishment of GNTES, that from the early years of the Revolution, sexual education was viewed as being critical to the country's overall development. In fact, almost immediately after GNTES was established, sexuality was re-defined as being important to one's health and well-being, and safe, responsible sex was viewed as being only achievable through education.

It is also important to consider how the understanding of sexual education differs in Cuba. Unlike many developed countries, such as Canada, the United States or the United Kingdom that view sexual education as what one learns in school classrooms, in Cuba it is understood as a broader concept. Sexual education is an integrated form of education that one receives on sex and sexuality from school, doctors, family, friends, and the media. ProNes, now ProNess, developed and implemented by CENESEX, along with ministries such as MINED and MINSAP, sought to develop sexual education from various approaches in both the formal and informal spheres. This was translated into a strategy that was able to communicate pertinent information to much, if not all, of the population. Rather than being restricted to school classrooms, sexual education became a constant, pervading all layers of Cuban society.

These different avenues of sexual education invariably promoted health and increasingly incorporated sexual diversity. From the 1990s, CENESEX's work has been significant in this regard. The Center's campaigns, networks, awareness-building, books, pamphlets, debates and work with other ministries and organizations have employed a strategy of sexual education that focuses on two themes: firstly, that sexuality is important to well-being; and secondly that sexual diversity should not be discriminated against. The importance of these themes is that they both promote the normalization of sexual diversity on the basis of health. Instead of being viewed as an independent entity, sexual education has been consistently understood as a critical way of contributing to individual and national health.

As a result of CENESEX efforts, the medical field has been promoting the normalization of sexual diversity, albeit at times unintentionally, or even reluctantly. As the discrimination-health link was cemented during the 1990s as a result of the threat of the spread of HIV/AIDS, medical professionals produced booklets that depicted sexual diversity as normal, while training has incorporated courses on the specific health needs of non-heteronormative sexual groups, and ProNess incorporated sexual diversity into its curricula. Finally, it is telling that CENESEX, the critical element in the evolutionary process, is itself a respected MINSAP center.

As has been demonstrated, the central theme underpinning the normalization of sexual diversity in revolutionary Cuba is undoubtedly health. The fundamental belief that discrimination is detrimental to health on an individual and a national level was the critical component of this process and of the development strategy. *Health* was thus the strategy through which Cuba was able to overcome its rooted prejudice and homophobia, and incorporate sexual diversity into the Revolution.

Health was the strategy through which human rights were obtained and promoted, rather than *vice versa*.

This particular strategy was developed and employed as a result of the country's relationship with, and understanding of, health and healthcare. Although, in the early years of the Revolution, both health and healthcare were developed largely out of the necessity to support production efforts, they soon evolved considerably and were viewed as important, for reasons of morality, equality, and *humanismo*. The importance that the Cuban government and population have placed on health and healthcare therefore allowed a space in which respect for sexual diversity could develop. In effect, placing sexual diversity within a health framework, whereby sexuality was correlated with well-being and national health rates, allowed it to engage with the specific qualities of the Cuban healthcare system and its understanding of health. Morality, equality, and *humanismo*, values produced and maintained by the population and government, ultimately initiated and later encouraged the normalization of sexual diversity.

For political reasons, the Cuban government did not receive any World Bank or IMF loans and thus was not required to institute Structural Adjustment Programs (SAPs); nor would the revolutionary government ever agree to do so. This made revolutionary Cuba one of the few developing countries that were not required by international loan stipulations to privatize education and healthcare, as well as institute other market-based reforms. As a result, education and healthcare were consistently provided by the state. Healthcare in particular was not altered to fit neoliberal market-forces, and specifically privatization. In a similar vein, the influence on the Cuban healthcare system of international NGOs or governments was very limited. In this context, while the Cuban system received information and financial assistance from other governments and NGOs, such as the IPPF, and some considerable support from international organizations such as the UN, it was largely under Cuban direction. The revolutionary medical system maintained its independence from significant external influences. The Cuban government and populace's views on health and healthcare were thus able to evolve more organically, resistant to the external pressures often experienced elsewhere.

Moreover, a change in attitudes toward sexual diversity in Cuba was not directed by a "strong state," but rather by the implementation of a community-based participatory model. State structures, such as the mass organizations and ministries, as well as members of the general population worked together to develop sexual education and sexual health. The product of their respective efforts was an ongoing normalization process through a negotiative model. Attitudes toward sexual diversity in revolutionary Cuba thus evolved through a series of specific Cuban circumstances. This resulted in the founding of CENESEX—a Cuban solution to a Cuban problem.

That said, although this is a uniquely Cuban strategy, it has significant value as a development approach. While the specific strategy itself cannot be copied and transplanted anywhere, aspects of it could be used to develop sexual diversity rights elsewhere. First, this study highlights the importance of education, in both the formal and informal spheres—information gained from ProNes, family doctors and the media, among others. National debate was ignited based on education needs and demands, as well as the publication of an enormous amount of information on sex and sexuality. For nearly six decades, education was not simply a means of informing the population, but rather served as a means of fuelling an ongoing public debate, through which attitudes and policies could evolve.

Secondly, debate is crucial. National debate, or public debate, allows opinions to be communicated, argued, and developed. In Cuba, the spaces for debate were both formal (such as FMC meetings), as well as informal. For sexual diversity these debates were central to the normalization process, and continue to be a significant means of attitudinal change at the individual, community, and national levels. This could undoubtedly be difficult for many cultures or regions, particularly those that have been vehemently anti-sexual diversity, however, as the Cuban case demonstrates, a small discussion can turn into a national debate.

Finally, and most importantly, what can be learned from this case is a greater understanding of a health-based approach, and by extension, the limitations of taking a strictly human rights-based approach to normalizing sexual diversity. While interpretations of human rights are malleable and often subjective across different cultures, by contrast health is important to all individuals and governments. Specifically in terms of development strategies, a health-based approach can be used to achieve enhanced human rights, while also improving health conditions. Based on Cuba's success, health can be used to alter opinions, as well as implement and direct change. This strategy provides an opportunity for a new and effective approach that could undoubtedly be used to create meaningful change elsewhere.

From this study, it can also be concluded that the development of CENESEX and the normalization of sexual diversity are also revealing of the Revolution. The Center's evolution and the changes in attitudes toward sexual diversity challenge the widely understood contention that revolutionary Cuba is an unalterable monolithic structure directed strictly by the government. While scholars have often employed the expression "Castro's Cuba," or similar comparable terminology, to discuss the Revolution, CENESEX's development suggests the precise opposite. As Kapcia's (2008; 2014) work asserts, rather than the government specifically directing change, instead change was implemented through a complex process of negotiation, reflecting a very different understanding of a previously held view of institutionalized immovability. In effect, this study illustrates that the understanding of "Castro's Cuba," led by a familial dictatorship, is false and must be updated.

In particular, what this complex evolution illustrates is the importance of this negotiative process when examining any component of the Revolution. Analysis of the evolution of attitudes toward sexual diversity, for example, illustrates the importance of the involvement and input of individuals, groups, and organizations in the implementation of change. For, as we have seen, the normalization of sexual diversity began as a result of needs expressed by women to the FMC regarding sexual education. The FMC independently established GNTES in 1972, five years before the state formally recognized and (re)established the group. GNTES and the FMC worked with various other elements of the Revolution's structure, such as the UJC, and numerous ministries, such as MINED, MINCULT, MINSAP to develop ProNes and institute change. The government and population's understanding of sexual education as a broad concept was paramount in this, as everyone from family doctors and teachers to community development specialists participated in its implementation, and are currently responsible for the implementation of ProNess throughout the island. The recent changes that have occurred as a result of CENESEX, such as celebrations for the International Day Against Homophobia, have also resulted from considerable effort by the state as well as the general population.

The importance of the negotiative approach within the evolutionary process is also highlighted by the role of national debate, which has remained a considerable factor throughout. It was present in the FMC's Congresses from the early 1960s, when they demanded improved sexual education, to discussions over the first popular-science book that incorporated discussion of homosexuality as "normal." National debate was responsible for incorporating sexuality, a previously taboo subject particularly for women, into public discourse, which in turn allowed a space for discussion of sexual diversity. These national debates are ongoing, as illustrated by the New Family Code, which in 2017 remained on the table in the National Assembly discussions. This view is further supported by Castro Espín's 2013 election into the National Assembly. It was well-known that her work focused on sexual diversity rights, a controversial topic, yet she was voted into a significant position of leadership with the understanding that she would continue efforts to normalize sexual diversity within the political structure.

As the study demonstrates, the normalization of sexual diversity did not occur as a result of the government's explicit work in the area. The revolutionary leaders did not decide at some stage that, due to national health, it was important to integrate non-heteronormative citizens into the national identity. Although Castro Espín would be discussed as one of the "Castros" in "Castro's Cuba," it is clear from the evolution of CENESEX in particular that this classic interpretation must be revisited. The Center and its specialists undoubtedly pushed the boundaries of what was, or should be, considered "revolutionary," and did so by working through a negotiative process.

Indeed an analysis of sexual diversity forces an examination that has been overlooked by others. This process suggests that a new understanding of the Cuban Revolution is needed. It should no longer be understood as a closed political system, but should instead be viewed as a complex process of negotiation. We have seen that it is not an unmovable, restrictive structure; rather, it is a multifaceted and dynamic system that is consistently in a stage of evolution. The process called "the Revolution" works and continues to evolve because of people and debate. It is consistently changing, adapting to fit contemporary needs. Change resulted from an evolutionary process of adjusting to needs and restrictions; it was a series of "push and pull" factors employed by various competing revolutionary elements and structures. These included political, cultural, and societal factors that collaborated to develop the necessary modifications to meet the demands of a given period.

The former United Nations Secretary-General, Ban Ki-moon, described the work of CENESEX as "magnificent." Following a visit to the Center in January 2014, he noted that, "to solve any problem, we must recognize that there is a problem—not hide or minimize it" (UN News 2014). The Cuban government and population identified homophobia as detrimental to health and well-being, and sought to correct it. It was not minimized, but instead recognized as a considerable problem within the Revolution, and corresponding efforts were made through various channels to change it.

Beyond the Revolution, the role of CENESEX is pivotal as it highlights the possibility of improving attitudes toward sexual diversity globally. If a country with a strong history of homophobia can change to receive international accolades for its efforts to promote rights, surely there is some significant value in its approach. Yet while considerable achievements have been made, it remains an ongoing process, as CENESEX continues to work to improve the lives of many of the island's citizens who still suffer from discrimination and prejudice because of their sexual orientation. Some problems persist, such as the legalization of the New Family Code, an increase in reported hate crimes, and criticism over ongoing discrimination. Nonetheless CENESEX will continue to try to meet these challenges, as its central aim of normalizing sexual diversity is pushed forward. As a cab driver in Havana explained on a recent trip, the work of CENESEX is important because it is "the right thing to do."

Appendices

Appendix A: List of Interviews

Name	*Position and Role*	*Interview Date*
Carolina Aguilar Ayerra	Carolina Aguilar Ayerra is one of the founders of the FMC, working closely with Yolanda Ferrer and Vilma Espín, among others. As a trained journalist, she worked for the FMC in publishing, editing dozens of books and hundreds of magazines, and remains heavily involved in the organization.	18 February 2013. CENESEX. Havana.
Mariela Castro Espín	Mariela Castro Espín is a trained child psychologist, with a Masters in Sexology and a PhD in Sociology (her thesis focused on transgender citizens). She is the director of CENESEX and SOCUMES, as well as a member of the National Assembly, and is involved with various national and international organizations that focus on themes regarding gender, sexuality, sexual education, and sexual health. She has published extensively, primarily on sexual diversity rights and sexual education in Cuba	30 January 2013. CENESEX. Havana.
Yasmany Díaz Figueroa	A psychologist with a Masters in Sexology, Díaz Figueroa worked at CENESEX in various capacities, particularly as the coordinator of the	28 January 2013. CENESEX. Havana.

Name	Position and Role	Interview Date
	Youth Network while this research was being carried out. He has also published sexual educational material for young people.	
Rosa Mayra Rodríguez Lauzurique	Rosa Mayra Rodríguez Lauzurique is a psychologist with a Masters in Sexology, and works at CENESEX in many capacities. She is the coordinator of the Transgender Network, and has published widely on themes of sexual education and sexual health, particularly regarding transgender persons.	20 February 2013. CENSEX. Havana.
Ada Caridad Alfonso Rodríguez	Ada Caridad Alfonso Rodríguez has served as interim director of CENESEX, as well as sub-director. She has been working at the Center in various capacities as a psychiatrist, and is the coordinator of the Women's Network. She has published extensively on the impact of issues related to sexual diversity, sexual violence, and STIs on mental health and well-being	29 Janaury 2013. CENESEX. Havana.
Marta María Ramírez	Marta María Ramírez is a social communications representative and reporter who has been working for CENESEX for some years. She has worked extensively on the Center's website, participated in public engagements, and has reported on many of the Center's activities.	4 February 2013. CENESEX. Havana.
Manuel Vázquez Seijido	Manuel Vázquez Seijido works as the Head of the Legal Advice at CENESEX.	13 February 2013. CENESEX. Havana.

Name	*Position and Role*	*Interview Date*
	In addition to his legal work at the Center and involvement in legal organizations throughout the country that focus on sexual diversity rights, he is also the coordinator of the CENESEX's Jurist Network.	
Pedro Pablo Valle Artiz	Pedro Pablo Valle Artiz is a renowned doctor, who has worked at CENESEX for several years. He practiced medicine at the Center, as well as participates in many of the Center's academic aspects, such as debates and panels. He was also the coordinator of the Men's Network while this research was being carried out, and worked closely with the Center on the *Jornada Contra la Homofobia*.	29 January 2013. CENSEX. Havana.

Appendix B: Statistical Analysis of Themes Examined in *Sexología y Sociedad* articles, 1994–2015

	Young People	*Abortions*	*Male sexuality*	*Fem. sexuality*	*Mature Gen.*	*Com. Dev.*	*Sex. Violence*	*Mention LGBT*	*LGBT*
1994	27%	27%	9%			27.3%			
1995	20%		7%	10%	7%	20%		2.5%	
1996	20%	10%	20%	15%	10%	10%		10%	
1997	14%	9%	9%	9%		14%	14%	4%	5%
1998	15%	6%	9%	24%	3%	3%	6%		
1999	27%	9%		27%	18%	9%			
2000	16%		5%	16%	6%	22%	6%		6%
2001	14%		14%	14%				14%	14%
2002	13%		20%	20%		13%	13%		7%
2003	10%		5%	15%	5%	10%	10%	21%	5%
2004	19%		5%	14.3%	5%	14%	9%	5%	19%
2005	25%			31%			6%	18%	6%
2006	12%		12%	20%	6%				6%
2007	7%	7%		38%		15%	7%		7%
2008	11%			22%		11%	11%		33%
2009	7%			23%	7%			23%	7%
2010			12%	12%	12%		12%	12%	12%
2011				14%		7%	7%	35%	14%
2012			60%			10%		20%	30%
2013	15%		8%	8%					38%
2014	12%		6%	6%			31%	6%	6%
2015	24%		6%				29%		35%

Timeline

Important Events in the Normalization of Sexual Diversity

1882 One of the earliest known court cases of discrimination against sexual diversity, a case entitled "Criminal proceedings against Mrs Enriqueta Fávez for disguising herself as a man by wearing a suit in order to trick Mrs Juana de León whom she legally married."

1888 One of the earliest known examples of discrimination against sexual diversity in the Cuban press, an article titled "Los maricones," published on the first page of the newspaper *La Cebolla*.

1960 The FMC was established.

1961 The "Night of the Three Ps," the round-up of "pederasts, prostitutes and pimps."

1962 The FMC's 1st National Congresses emphasized the need for comprehensive sexual education.

1965 MINSAP report noted that there is no known biological cause of homosexuality and theorized that homosexuality was a learned behavior.

1965 Research began on how to correct homosexuality.

1965–1968 The UMAP camps used for "re-education."

1966 UNEAC held emergency meeting to defend and support their colleagues, demanding that they not be sent to UMAP camps.

1969 Deputy Minister of Education Abel Prieto Morales published article entitled "Homosexualismo" in *Bohemia*.

1971–1976 The *Quinquenio Gris* cultural repression.

1971 First National Congress on Education and Culture, which banned homosexuals from participating in the educational process and promoted the need for comprehensive sexual education.

1972 The National Group for Work on Sexual Education (GNTES) was established by Vilma Espín and Celestino Álvarez Lajonchere.

1974 Law 1267 established, which outlined the restrictions on homosexuals, including prohibiting them from working in any position in which they could influence children or young people.

1975 The Family Code was introduced, which challenged previously held views of gender roles.

1975 The PCC's 1st Congress, at which the Commission On the Attention to Infancy, Youth, and the Equality of Rights of Women with the principal aim of publishing sexual education material was formally established (referred to as either la Comisión Permanente de la Asamblea Nacional del Poder Popular "Sobre la atención a la infancia y la igualdad de derechos de la mujer," or the "Comisión Permanente para la Atención a la Infancia, la Juventud, y la Igualdad de Derechos de la Mujer").

1977 The government formally recognized and legitimated the FMC's GNTES.

1979 GNTES published East German sexologist Siegfried Schnabl's *Man and Woman in Intimacy*, the last chapter of which centered on the need to respect sexual diversity (reprinted in 1985 and a second edition was published in 1989).

1979 Homosexual acts between adults in private is de-criminalized in an amendment to the Penal Code.

1979 Following requests from the FMC, MINSAP authorized the establishment of a specialized multidisciplinary team led by GNTES, which would provide comprehensive assistance to transgender citizens.

1980 Mariel boatlift, in which many Cubans pretended to be homosexual in order to be more undesirable by the revolutionary government and thus more likely to be able to leave for the United States.

1980 The 2nd PCC Congress re-emphasized the need for improved sexual education, and GNTES is noted as being the representative group of the Comisión Permanente de la Asamblea Nacional del Poder Popular "Sobre la atención a la infancia y la igualdad de derechos de la mujer."

1980 3rd FMC Congress, which further emphasized the need for improved sexual education.

1981 Vilma Espín became the president of the Comisión Permanente de la Asamblea Nacional del Poder Popular "Sobre la atención a la infancia y la igualdad de derechos de la mujer," and the FMC assumed further control over the development of sexual education.

1981 Siegfried Schnabl's book entitled *En defensa de amor* was published (and re-printed in 1985), which also supported the need to respect sexual diversity.

1981 Heinrich Brückner's book entitled *¿Piensas ya en el amor?*, which discussed homosexuality as deviant behavior, was published (reprinted in 1985).

1985 GNTES formed the Cuban Multidisciplinary Society for the Study of Sexuality (SOCUMES).

1985 GNTES coordinator Monika Krause's book entitled *Algunos temas fundamentales sobre educación sexual*, which discussed the importance of sexual education and respect for sexuality, was published (reprinted in 1987 and 1988).

1987 GNTES coordinator Monika Krause's book entitled *Educación sexual. Selección de lecturas,* in which significant members of GNTES noted the importance of sexual education, was published (reprinted in 1988).

1988 MINSAP minister signed resolution to change GNTES into the National Center of Sexual Education (CENESEX).

1989 CENESEX is officially established under the auspices of MINSAP.

1990 The World Health Organization removes homosexuality from the list of known mental illnesses.

1992 In an interview with Tomás Borge, Fidel Castro noted that he was opposed to all forms of discrimination, including that related to homosexuality.

1993 The film *Fresa y chocolate* is released.

1994 CENESEX began publishing the research journal *Sexología y Sociedad.*

2003–2004 CENESEX shifted its focus to emphasize respect for sexual diversity.

2003 CENESEX's Women's Network was established, focusing on health needs of sexually diverse women.

2005 CENESEX, with the support of MINSAP, re-established GNTES' Multidisciplinary Commission that sought to assist transgender people as the National Commission for the Integral Care of Transsexuals.

2006 Cuba participated in the "Gay Olympics" in Montreal, Canada.

2007 CENESEX participated for the first time in the International Day Against Homophobia.

2008 CENESEX, along with other Cuban elements, such as the Ministry of Culture, celebrated the International Day Against Homophobia in Havana (known as the *Jornada contra la homophobia*).

2008 *Bohemia* published an article that focuses on the importance of respecting sexual diversity for the first time.

2008 Public Health Minister signed Resolution 126, which authorized the creation of a center that would provide comprehensive healthcare for transsexuals, including free gender-reassignment surgeries, medication, and therapy.

2010 At the United Nations General Assembly's Social, Humanitarian and Cultural Affairs Committee, Cuban diplomats voted in favor of an amendment that would replace any reference to "sexual orientation" with the more general expression "discriminatory reason on any basis."

2010 Fidel Castro personally apologized for the UMAP camps, assuming full responsibility.

2011 CENESEX's Men's Network (Men for Diversity) was founded, focusing on normalizing sexual diversity through awareness-building.

2011 The PCC changes its Fundamental Principals to incorporate sexual diversity.

2012 CENESEX's Youth Network was established, focusing on normalizing sexual diversity through consciousness-raising among young people.

2012 CENESEX's Transgender Network was established, focusing on normalizing sexual diversity through awareness-building, and proving support for the transgender community.

2012 Cuba's first transgender woman was elected at the municipal government level.

2012 The New Family Code is formally presented to the National Assembly.

2013 CENESEX's Jurist Network was established, focusing on promoting respect for sexual diversity through changes in legislation.

2013 The new Labour Code was released to the public and prompts debate, as it does not make specific mention to discrimination on the basis of sexual orientation or gender identity.

2013 SEXSALUD is launched at the University of Medical Sciences of Santiago de Cuba.

2014 The celebrations for the International Day Against Homophobia occurred in seven of Cuba's fifteen provinces, and incorporated international and national specialists from multidisciplinary backgrounds.

Bibliography

Acosta, Dalia. 2006. "Nueva Propuesta sobre diversidad sexual." *Cultura y Sociedad* 1 (January).

———. 2008. "Health-Cuba: Free Sex Change Operations Approved." *IPS*, June 6. Accessed June 22, 2014. http://www.ipsnews.net/2008/06/health-cuba-free-sex-change-operations-approved.

———. 2009a. "Homophobia is Not Incurable." *IPS*, June 6. Accessed May 22, 2014. http://www.cuba-l.com/homophobia-is-not-incurable.

———. 2009b. "Machismo gay y violencia." *SEMlac*, May 22. Accessed June 22, 2014. http://diversidad.redsemlac-cuba.net/Sociedad/Machismo-gay-y-violencia.html.

———. 2010a. "Cuba: Foreign Ministry Explains Controversial 'Sexual Orientation' Vote to Activists." *IPS*, December 2. Accessed February 2, 2012. http://www.lexisnexis.com:80/uk/nexis/results/docview/docview.do?start=29&sort=BOOLEAN&format=GNBFI&risb=21_T13960687041.

———. 2010b. "Cuba: Lesbians Demand Fair Treatment from Health Providers." *IPS*, November 26. Accessed June 22, 2014. http://www.ipsnews.net/2010/11/cuba-lesbians-demand-fair-treatment-from-health-providers/.

———. 2010c. "'Cuba: Sexual Orientation' Vote in UN Panel Kicks up Controversy." *IPS*, December 1. Accessed February 2, 2012. http://www.lexisnexis.com/80/uk/nexis/results/docview/docview.do?start=30&sort=BOOLEAN&format=GNBFI&risb=21_T13960687041.

———. 2011a. "Ataque a la homofobia." *IPS*, May 3. Accessed September 20, 2014. http://www.ipsnoticias.net/2011/05/cuba-ataque-a-la-homofobia/.

———. 2011b. "Cuba: Diversidad sexual en ciudad machista." *IPS*, May 18. Accesed May 10, 2011. http://www.ipsnoticias.net/2011/05/cuba-diversidad-sexual-en-ciudad-machista/.

Aguilar Ayerra, Carolina. 2013. Interview with Emily J. Kirk. February 18. Havana.

Aguilera Ribeaux, Daisy. 2001. "Introducción." *Violencia contra la Mujer: Un problema de todos y todas. Recuentos y Propuestas*. 20–36. Havana: CENESEX.

Aguirre, B.E. 1994. "The Conventionalization of Collective Behavior in Cuba." *American Journal of Sociology* 90 (3): 541–66.

Alfonso Fraga, Juan Carlos. 1994. "Fecundidad y aborto en la adolescencia: Algunas Carácterísticas." *Sexología y Sociedad* 1 (0): 8–9.

Alfonso Rodríguez, Ada Caridad. 2007. *Violencia contra la mujer: Una alerta para profesonales de la salud*. Havana: Editorial CENESEX, with the support of the Sistema de Naciones Unidas en Cuba, and the Fondo de Desarrollo de Las Naciones Unidas para la Mujer (UNIFEM).

———. 2013. Interview with Emily J. Kirk. January 29. Havana.

Alfonso Rodríguez, Ada C., Elvia de Dios Blanco, Ivón Ernand Thames, and Rosa Mayra Rodríguez Lauzurique. 2008a. *Diversidad sexual, salud mental y VIH: Temas para el trabajo con poblaciones clave*. Havana: Editorial CENESEX.

Alfonso Rodríguez, Ada Caridad, Magaly González Jiménez, and Rosa Mayra Rodríguez Lauzurique. 2008b. *Género, ITS y VIH: Cuestiones básicas para la prevención. Cartilla de apoyo para el trabajo de las comisiones de educación sexual*. Havana: Editorial CENESEX.

Alfonso Rodríguez, Ada Caridad, and Magaly González Jiménez. 2009. *Prevenir HIV a diario. Definiciones útiles en la producción de salud sexual*. Havana: Editorial Cenesex.

AllAfrica.com. 2012. "OIG Diagnostic Review Says Cuba Can Be a Model for Other Countries." May 28. Accessed September 10, 2014. http://allafrica.com/stories/201205281226.html.

Álvarez Carril, Elcida and Damaris Álvarez Zapata. 1995. "SIDA ¿Qué opinan los niños." *Sexología y Sociedad* 1 (3): 38–39.

Álvarez Lajonchere, Celestino. 1994. "El aborto en Cuba, aspectos jurídicos y médico-sociales." *Sexología y Sociedad* 1 (0): 6–7.

———. 1996. "Educación sexual en Cuba. Reseña histórica." *Sexología y Sociedad* 2 (6): 25–29.

Anderson, Benedict. 1983. *Imagined Communities*. London: Verso.

Ansa Latina Roma. 2011. "Cuba: Piden "desarticular" discriminación sexual." May 8. Accessed September 20, 2014. http://www.cuba-l.com/cuba-piden-quotdesarticular quot-discriminacion-sexual/.

Antiproyecto de Ley Código de Trabajo. 2013. Accessed July 14, 2014. http://www.granma.cu/granmad/Anteproyecto-Ley-Codigo-TRabajo-Cuba-2013.pdf.

Arenas, Reinaldo. 2001. *Before Night Falls*. Translated by the Estate of Reinaldo Arenas and Dolores M. Koch. London: Serpent's Tail.

Arguelles, Lourdes and Ruby B. Rich. 1984. "Homosexuality, homophobia, and Revolution: Notes toward an understanding of the Cuban lesbian and gay male experience, part I." *Signs* 9 (4): 683–99.

———. 1985. "Homosexuality, Homophobia, and Revolution: Notes toward an Understanding of the Cuban Lesbian and Gay Male Experience, Part II." *Signs* 11 (1): 120–36.

Arreola, Gerardo. 2006. "El tema de la bisexualidad polariza a Cuba." *La Jornada*, May 8. Accessed June 22, 2014. http://www.walterlippmann.com/lgbt-cuba007.html.

———. 2008. "Cuba celebrará por segunda vez la jornada mundial contra la homofobia." *La Jornada*, May 6. Accessed May 6, 2014. http://www.jornada.unam.mx/2008/05/06/index.php?section=mundo&article=029n2mun.

Arrue Hernándes, María Imilse. 2005. *¿Cómo demuestro que te amo? Programa para la formación de promotores y promotoras adolescentes de salud sexual con énfasis en la prevención de ITS-VIH/SIDA*. Havana: Editorial CENESEX.

Artiles de León, Ileana, Ana María. Cano López, Mariela Castro Espín, Carolina Díaz Bravo and Mérida López. *Mi proyecto de vida*. Pamphlet. Editorial Pueblo y Educación. Havana. Undated.

Asamblea Nacional de Poder Popular. 1995. Constitución de la República de Cuba. Havana: Gaceta Oficial de la República de Cuba.

Avendaño, Bárbara. 2008. "Diversidad sexual: Desafiando molinos." *Bohemia* 11 (11): 24–28.

Baksh-Soodeen, Rawwida. 1998. "Issues of difference in contemporary Caribbean feminism." *Feminist Review* 159: 74–85.

Ball, Carlos A. 2010. From the closet to the courtroom: Five LGBT rights lawsuits that have changed our nation. Boston: Beacon Press.

Bandarage, Asoka. 1984. "Women in Development: Liberalism, Marxism, Marxism-Feminism." *Development and Change* 15 (4): 495–515.

Baron, Guy. 2011. *Gender in Cuban cinema from the modern to the postmodern*. Oxford: Peter Lang.

Barrett, Michèle. 1980. *Women's Oppression Today: Problems in Marxist Feminist Analysis*. London: Verso.

Basham, Richard. 1976. "Machismo." *Frontiers: A Journal of Women Studies* 1 (2): 126–43.

BBC. 2013. "Cubans March Against Homophobia in Havana." May 12. Accessed September 20, 2014. http://www.bbc.co.uk/news/world-latin-america-22497436.

Bejel, Emilio. 2001. *Gay Cuban Nation*. Chicago: The University of Chicago Press.

Bengelsdorf, Carollee. 1997. "Terreno en debate: La mujer en Cuba. Un ensayo bibliográfico." *Temas* 9 (January-March): 121–31.

Bhavnani, Kum-Kum and Margaret Coulson. 1986. "Socialist-Feminism: Out of the Blue." *Feminist Review* 23: 81–89.

Bohemia. 1987a. "Educación sexual: Tradiciones y costumbres anacrónicas." 79 (15): 56–57.
———. 1987b. "Embarazo en la adolescencia: Epidemia de alta frecuencia." 79 (26): 21–25.
———. 1987c. "Televisión y el sexo." 79 (30): 84.
———. 2001a. "Embarazo en la adolescencia." 93 (25): 27–32.
———. 2001b. "Hablar de sexualidad a su hijo." 93 (24): 69.
———. 2001c. "La vitamina sexual." 93 (15): 69.
———. 2001d. "Prisioneros del sexo." 93 (19): 69.
———. 2001e. "Relaciones sexuales." 93 (26): 69.
———. 2008. "Diversidad sexual: Desafiando molinos." 100 (12): 24–28.
Bonilla, Laura. 2007. "Once persecuted, gays find Cuba more tolerant." *AFP*, January 21. Accessed June 22, 2014. http://www.caribbeannetnews.com/cgi-script/csArticles/articles/000052/005285.htm.
Bowry, Gill. 1989. "Lesbians in Cuba." *Off Our Back* 19 (3): 6–7.
Bravo, Ernesto. 1998. *Development within Underdevelopment?: New Trends in Cuban Medicine*. Havana: Editorial José Martí.
Brown, Sarah. 1988. "Feminism, International Theory and International Relations of Gender Inequality." *Millennium: Journal of International Studies* 17 (3): 461–75.
Browne, Katherine and Catherine J. Nash. 2014. "Resisting LGBT Rights Where 'We Have Won': Canada and Great Britain." *Journal of Human Rights* 13 (3): 322–36.
Brückner, Heinrich. 1980a. *Antes de que nazca un niño*. 2nd ed. Havana: Gente Nueva.
———. 1980b. *Cuando tu hijo te pregunta*. 2nd ed. Havana: Gente Nueva.
———. 1981. *¿Piensas ya en el amor?* Havana: Gente Nueva. Havana.
Cabezas, Amalia L. 2009. *Economies of Desire: Sex Tourism in Cuba and the Dominican Republic*. Philadelphia: Temple University Press.
CAME. 1981. *La mujer en la sociedad socialista*. Moscow: Consejo de Ayuda Mutua Económica Secretariado.
Cano López, Ana María. 2009. *Programa Aprender a Prevenir: Manual de Actualización*. Havana: Editorial CENESEX.
Casal, Lourdes. 1975. "Images of Cuban Society Among Pre- and Post-Revolutionary Novelists." PhD diss., New School of Social Research.
Castillo, Raisa Rambaut, José Joanes Fiol, and Jaime Pintos Valluerca. 1999. "Characteristics of the HIV/AIDS Epidemic in a Prison Survey Group." *Cuban Medical Research*. Accessed November 4, 2012. http://www.medicc.org/publications/medicc_review/III/hiv-aids/pages/characteristics.
Castro Espín, Mariela. 1995. "Preguntas prohibidas." *Sexología y Sociedad* 1 (1): 22–24.
———. 2003. *¿Qué nos pasa en la pubertad?* Havana: Editorial Pueblo y Educación.
———. 2004. "De la Habana a Montreal." *Sexología y Sociedad* 10 (25): 4–5.
———. 2007. "Carta de la directora." *Sexología y Sociedad* 13 (33): 3.
———. 2008a. "La atención a transexuales en Cuba y su inclusión en las políticas sociales." *Sexología y Sociedad* 14 (36): 4–10.
———. 2008b. "La atención a transexuales en Cuba y su inclusión en las políticas sociales." In *La Transexualidad en Cuba*, edited by Mariela Castro Espín, 15–43. Havana: Centro Nacional de Educación Sexual.
———. 2009. "Carta de la directora: Vigésimo aniversario de CENESEX." *Sexología y Sociedad* 15 (41): 3.
———. 2010. "Declaración de la SOCUMES y el CENESEX sobre voto de Cuba en la Asamblea General de las Naciones Unidas." CENESEX. November 24.
———. 2011. "A Cuban Policy Approach to Sex Education." *Cuban Studies* 42: 23–34.
———. 2013. Interview with Emily J. Kirk. January 30. Havana.
Castro, Fidel. 1961. "Palabras a los intelectuales." Havana: Consejo Nacional de Cultura.
———. 1963a. "Fidel en el Acto Conmemorativo del 27 de noviembre, celebrado en la escalinata de la Universidad de La Habana, el 27 de noviembre de 1963." Accessed September 20, 2014 http://www.cuba.cu/gobierno/discursos/1963/esp/f271163e.html

———. 1963b. "Fidel en la clausura del X Congreso Médico y Estomatólogico Nacional, el 24 de febrero de 1963." Accessed September 20, 2014 http://www.cuba.cu/gobierno/discursos/1963/esp/f240263e.html.

———. 1964. "Fidel en el acto de graduación de 250 médicos, celebrado en el teatro de la CTC Revolucionaria, el 10 de septiembre de 1964." Accessed September 20, 2014. http://www.cuba.cu/gobierno/discursos/1964/esp/f100964e.html.

———. 1969. "Fidel en la inauguración del policlínico del Valle del Perú, en Jaruco, el 8 de enero de 1969." Accessed September 20, 2014. http://constitucionweb.blogspot.co.uk/2014/01/discurso-de-fidel-castro-en-la_8251.html.

———. 1978. "Fidel en el acto de inicio del Curso Escolar 1978-1979, efectuado en el Instituto Politécnico de la Salud de la provincia de Camaguey, el 4 de septiembre de 1978." Accessed September 20, 2014. http://www.cuba.cu/gobierno/discursos/1978/esp/f040978e.html.

———. 1980. "'No sería posible escribir la historia de nuestra revolución en los últimos 20 años sin la Federación de Mujeres Cubanas.' Discurso pronunciado por el comandante en jefe Fidel Castro Ruz, Primer Secretario del Comité Central del Partido Comunista de Cuba y Presidente de los Consejos de Estado y de Ministros, en la clausura del III Congreso de la Federación de Mujeres Cubanas, efectuado en el teatro 'Carlos Marx,' el 8 de Marzo de 1980, 'Año del Segundo Congreso.'" *Bohemia* 72 (11): 50–61.

———. 1992. *Un grano de maíz: Conversación con Tomás Borge*. Havana: Oficina de publicaciones del Consejo de Estado.

———. 1999. "Key address by Fidel Castro Ruz, President of the Republic of Cuba, at the inauguration of the Latin American School of Medicine." November 15. Accessed July 15, 2014. http://www.cuba.cu/gobierno/discursos/1999/ing/il51199i.html.

Castro, Raúl. 2012. "Discurso de Raúl Castro: 'El rumbo ya ha sido trazado.'" *Cubadebate*, January 29. Accessed June 22, 2014. http://www.cubadebate.cu/opinion/2012/01/29/discurso-de-raul-castro-en-la-primera-conferencia-nacional-del-pcc/#.U8PnAc3A3JF.

Centro Cultural Pablo de la Torriente Brau. 2012. "Exposición de cartels: NO a la violencia contra la mujer." Articularte Red. Pamphlet.

CENESEX. n.d. "Programa de educación para las escuelas de arte." Havana.

———. 2001. "Profesor Celestino Álvarez Lajonchere, evolución del eminente obstetra y salubrista cubano." *Sexología y Sociedad* 7 (17): 33–36.

———. 2005. "Código de ética para profesionales de la sexología en Cuba." *Sexología y Sociedad*. 11 (27): 27–31.

———. 2012a. "¿Quiénes Somos?" Accessed June 22, 2014. http://www.cenesex.org/quienes-somos/.

———. 2012b. "Red de Juristas por derechos sexuales. Documento Base."

———. 2013. "I Cónclave Nacional Virtual de Estudiantes Universitarios vinculados al estudio de la Sexualidad, SEXSALUD 2013." January 28. Accessed June 22, 2014. http://www.cenesex.org/eventos/i-conclave-nacional-virtual-de-estudiantes-universitarios-vinculados-al-estudio-de-la-sexualidad-sexsalud%C2%B42013/.

———. 2014a. "Red de Jóvenes por la Salud y los Derechos Sexuales." Accessed June 22, 2014. http://ensentidocontrario.com/13524/celebran-jornadas-sobre-salud-transexual-en-cuba/.

———. 2014b. "Red de Juristas por derechos sexuales." Accessed June 22, 2014. http://www.cenesex.org/redes-sociales-comunitarias/.

———. 2014c. "Red de Mujeres Lesbianas y Bisexuales." Accessed June 22, 2014. http://ensentidocontrario.com/13524/celebran-jornadas-sobre-salud-transexual-en-cuba/.

———. 2014d. "Red de personas Transgénero (Trans Cuba)." Accessed June 22, 2014. http://ensentidocontrario.com/13524/celebran-jornadas-sobre-salud-transexual-en-cuba/.

———. 2014e. "Red Humanidad por la Diversidad (HxD)." Accessed June 22, 2014. http://ensentidocontrario.com/13524/celebran-jornadas-sobre-salud-transexual-en-cuba/.

Chávez Negrín, Ernesto. 2011. "La violencia en las familias cubanas analizada por las investigaciones sociales." In *Violencia familiar en Cuba. Estudios, realidades y desafíos sociales*, edited by Mareelén Díaz Tenorio, Alberta Durán Gondar, Yohanka Valdés Jiménez, Ernesto Chávez Negrín, Patricia Gazmuri Núñez, and Silvia Padrón Durán, 187–212. Havana: Publicaciones Acuario and Editorial CENESEX.

Chinchilla, Norma Stoltz. 1991. "Marxism, Feminism, and the Struggle for Democracy in Latin America." *Gender and Society* 5 (3): 291–310.

Collazo, Vivián. 2010. "Concluye en Cuba Congreso de Educación y Terapia Sexual." *Prensa Latina*, January 22. Accessed June 22, 2014. http://www.visionesalternativas.com/index.php?option=com_content&view=article&id=5748:concluye-en-cuba-congreso-de-educacion-y-terapia-sexual&catid=2.

Coll Sánchez, Gerardo. 1995. "Contraceptivos hormonales." *Sexología y Sociedad* 1 (2): 10–13.

Corrales, Javier. 2012. "LGBT Rights In The Americas." *Americas Quarterly* 6 (2): 88–94.

Correo del Orinoco. 2013. "Cuba celebrará VI Jornada contra la homofobia." March 25. Accessed May 19, 2014. http://www.correodelorinoco.gob.ve/multipolaridad/cuba-celebrara-vi-jornada-contra-homofobia/.

Coward, Rosalind. 1983. *Patriarchal Precedents: Sexuality and Social Relations*. London: Routledge.

Cubadebate. 2011. "Proyecto de documento base de la primera conferencia nacional del Partido Communista de Cuba." October 14. Accessed November 1, 2014. http://www.cubadebate.cu/noticias/2011/10/14/descargue-proyecto-de-documento-que-discutirá-conferencia-nacional-del-particdo-pdf/.

CubaSí. 2013a. "Adelantos de la VI Jornada contra la homofobia en Cuba." March 26. Accessed June 22, 2014. http://www.cubasi.cu/cubasi-noticias-cuba-mundo-ultima-hora/item/15662-adelantos-de-la-vi-jornada-contra-la-homofobia-en-cuba?device=desktop.

———. 2013b. "Celebrará Cuba VI Jornada contra la homofobia." March 25. Accessed June 22, 2014. http://www.cubasi.cu/cubasi-noticias-cuba-mundo-ultima-hora/item/15608-celebrara-cuba-vi-jornada-contra-la-homofobia?device=desktop.

d'Adesky, Anne-Christine. 2003. "Cuba Fights AIDS Its Own Way." *The Body*. Accessed January 10, 2016. http://www.thebody.com/content/art32967.html.

Daily Mail. 2011. "Transgender woman ties knot with gay man after having state-funded sex-change op." August 15. Accessed September 20, 2014. http://www.dailymail.co.uk/news/article-2025965/Transgender-woman-Ignacio-Estrada-marries-gay-man-LGBT-wedding-Cuba.html.

Danielson, Ross. 1985. "Medicine in the Community." In *Cuba: Twenty-Five Years of Revolution 1959–1984*, edited by Sandor Halebsky and John M. Kirk, 45–61. New York: Praeger.

de la Cuesta Freijomil, Dolores. 1997. "Hablemos francamente: ¿Participa el hombre en el embarazo?" *Mujeres*, March.

De la Cruz, Dania. 1980. *Movimiento Feminismo Cubano*. Havana: Editorial Política.

De la Osa, José A. 2010. "Infecciones de Transmisión Sexual/VIH/SIDA Tú puedes protegerte." *Granma*, July 13.

Díaz Álvarez, María Teresa. 2005. *Conserva tus sueños. Manual educativo para la formación de promotores y promotoras adolescentes*. Havana: Editorial CENESEX.

Díaz, Elaine. 2014. "Luces y sombras del nuevo código de trabajo cubano." *Global Voices*, June 15. Accessed June 15, 2015. http://es.globalvoicesonline.org/2014/06/25/luces-y-sombras-del-nuevo-codigo-de-trabajo-cubano/.

Díaz Figueroa, Yasmany. 2013. Interview with Emily J. Kirk. January 28. Havana.

Díaz Figueroa, Yasmany, Ada Caridad Alfonso Rodríguez and Zullendrys Kindelán Arias. 2010. *Adolescentes y jóvenes an la prevención de las ITS y el VIH. Manual de apoyo para promotores y promotoras*. Havana: Editorial CENESEX.

Díaz Noriega, Oscar, Wally Thompson Forbes. 1995. "La edad del erotismo: Sexualidad en la tercera edad." *Sexología y Sociedad* 1 (1): 14–17.

Díaz Tenorio, Marleenlén, Alberta Durán Gondar, Yohanka Valdés Jiménez, Ernesto Cávez Negrín, Ptracia Gazmuri Núñez and Silvia Padrón Durán. (2011). *Violencia familar en Cuba*. Havana: Editorial CENESEX.

Díaz Vallina, Alvira. 2001. "The Invisibility and Visibility of Women in the History of Cuba." In *Cuban Women: History, Contradictions and Contemporary Challenges*, edited by Colleen Lundy and Norma Vasallo Barrueta, 1–22. Ottawa: Carlton University Graphic Services.

Dunphy, Richard. 2000. *Sexual Politics*. Edinburgh: Edinburgh University Press.

Echarry, Irina. 2009. "Homophobia Is the Problem, Not Gays." *Havana Times*, May 19. Accessed May 19, 2014. http://www.havanatimes.org/?p=8922.

Ecodiario. 2012. "Cuba inicia jornada contra la homofobia que honrará a escritor Piñera." May 8. Accessed September 20, 2014. http://ecodiario.eleconomista.es/internacional/noticias/3951145/05/12/Cuba-inicia-jornada-contra-la-homofobia-que-honrara-a-escritor-Pinera.html.

Edith, Dixie and Helen H. Hormilla. 2009. "Entre hombres anda el virus." *Bohemia* 101 (7): 28–35.

Editorial de Ciencias Sociales. 1975. "History Will Absolve Me." Translated by Pedro Álvarez Tabío and Andrew Paul Boot. Havana. Accessed September 20, 2014. https://www.marxists.org/history/cuba/archive/castro/1953/10/16.htm.

EFE. 2008. "Cuba tiene más de 9.000 personas diagnosticadas con VIH/sida." May 10. Accessed June 22, 2014. http://www.emol.com/noticias/internacional/2008/05/10/303775/cuba-tiene-mas-de-9000-personas-diagnosticadas-con-vihsida.html.

———. 2013. "Grupo LGBT independiente recogerá firmas en Cuba." June 29. Accessed June 22, 2014. http://www.larioja.com/agencias/20130629/mas-actualidad/sociedad/grupo-lgbt-independiente-recogera-firmas_201306292345.html.

Egües Cantero, Gladys. 1997. "Hablemos francamente: Reflexiones sobre la crisis de la mediana edad." *Muejres*. No. 3: 13.

elEconomista.es. 2012. "Cuba inicia jornada contra la homofobia que honrará a escritor Piñera." May 8. Accessed June 22, 2014. http://ecodiario.eleconomista.es/internacional/noticias/3951145/05/12/Cuba-inicia-jornada-contra-la-homofobia-que-honrara-a-escritor-Pinera.html#.Kku8i9pMX2V25wF.

El Universo. 2012. "Cuba 'está lista' para el matrimonio gay, dice hija de Raúl Castro." December 10. Accessed September 20, 2012. http://www.eluniverso.com/2012/12/10/1/1361/cuba-esta-lista-matrimonio-gay-dice-hija-raul-castro.html.

Engels, Friedrich. 1972. *The Origins of the Family, Private Property and the State*. New York: International Publishers.

Epps, Brad. 1995. "Proper Conduct: Reinaldo Arenas, Fidel Castro, and the Politics of Homosexuality." *Journal of the History of Sexuality* 6 (2): 231–83.

Ernesto, Alejandro and Enrique de la Osa. 2011. "Protagonizan cubanos marcha contra la homofobia en La Habana." *Cubadebate*, May 14. Accessed May 17, 2014. http://www.cubadebate.cu/noticias/2011/05/14/protagonizan-cubanos-marcha-contra-la-homofobia-en-la-habana-fotos/#.U2exNMeTY7A.

Espín, Vilma, Asela de los Santos, and Yolanda Ferrer. 2012a. "It Gave us a Sense of Worth. Interview with Asela de los Santos." In *Women in Cuba: The Making of a Revolution Within the Revolution*, edited by Mary-Alice Waters, 53–115. New York: Pathfinder.

———. 2012b. "What It Meant to Be Female Began to Change. Interview with Yolanda Ferrer." In *Women in Cuba: The Making of a Revolution Within the Revolution*, edited by Mary-Alice Waters, 195–214. New York: Pathfinder.

———. 2012c. "With No Preconceived Structure or Agenda. Interview with Vilma Espín." In *Women in Cuba: The Making of a Revolution Within the Revolution*, edited by Mary-Alice Waters, 215–87. New York: Pathfinder.

Family Code. 1979. *Law No. 1289, of February 14, 1975, Official Gazette, February 15, 1975*. Havana: The Chamber of Commerce of the Republic of Cuba.

Farnós Morejón, Alfonso, Fernando González Quiñones, and Raúl Hernández Castellón. 1982. *Las mujeres trabajadoras y los cambios demograficos en Cuba*. Havana: Centro de Estudios Demográficos. Facultad de Economía, Universidad de la Habana.

Fee, Elizabeth. 1988. "Sex Education in Cuba: An Interview with Dr. Celestino Lajonchere." *International Journal of Health Services* 18 (2): 343–56.

Fernández Martínez, Marta and Yamila González Ferrer. (2008). "Una mirada jurídica de la transexulidad en Cuba." In *La transexualidad en Cuba*, edited by Mariela Castro Espín, 144–82. Havana: Centro Nacional De Educación Sexual.

Fiallo, Miguel A. 1995. "La nueva píldora." *Sexología y Sociedad* 1 (1): 7.

Figes, Eva. 1970. *Patriarchal Attitudes*. London: Faber and Faber.

Fink, Sheri. 2003. "Cuba's Energetic AIDS Doctor." *American Journal of Public Health* 93 (5): 712–16.

Firestone, Shulamith. 1970. *The dialectic of sex: The case of feminist revolution*. London: Jonathan Cape.

Flórez Madan, Lourdes. 1994. "La educación sexual en Cuba: Programa nacional." *Sexología y Sociedad* 1 (0): 22–27.

FMC. 1962. *1er Congreso Nacional. Federación de Mujeres Cubanas*. Havana: Ministerio de Industrias, Empresa Consolidada de Artes Gráficas.

———. 1973a. "Debates de Salud: El embarazo." *Mujeres* 12 (4): 62–63.

———. 1973b. "Debates de Salud: Hemorragias uterinas y postmenopaúsicas." *Mujeres* (13) 10: 62–63.

———. 1975. *Memoria: II Congreso Nacional de la Federación de Mujeres Cubanas*. Havana: Instituto Cubano del Libro, Editorial Orbe.

———. 1982. *Boletín FMC*. Havana: Federation of Cuban Women Empresa Editorial de la Mujer.

———. 1984a. *Memorias del 3er Congreso de la FMC*. Havana: Federación de Mujeres Cubanas, Editorial de Ciensias Sociales.

———. 1984b. "En defensa del amor." *Mujeres* 24 (2): 56–57.

———. 1987. *Memorias: Del IV Congreso de la Federación de Mujeres Cubanas*. Havana: Federación de Mujeres Cubanas and Editorial Política.

———. 1996. *La mujer en la Revolución y la Revolución en la mujer*. Edited by Carolina Aguilar Ayerra and Isabel Moya. Havana: Editorial de la Mujer.

———. 1997. "Arquitectas de su destino." *Mujeres* 1: 2–4.

———. 1998. *Realidades y desafíos. Encuentro internacional de solidaridad entre mujeres*. Havana: Editorial de la Mujer.

———. 2008. *Por Siempre Vilma*. Havana: Editorial de la Mujer.

Fone, Bryne. 2000. *Homophobia, A History*. New York: Metropolitan Books.

Formental Hernández, Soura; Iyamira Hernández Pita and Teresa Fernández De Juan. 2014. "Masculinities in Cuba: Description and Analysis of a Case Study from a Gender Perspective." *Masculinidades y cambio social* 3 (3): 220–47.

Foucault, Michel. 1990a. *A History of Sexuality Vol. 1: An Introduction*. London: Vintage Books.

———. 1990b. *A History of Sexuality Vol. 2: The Use of Pleasure*. London: Vintage Books.

———. 1990c. *A History of Sexuality Vol. 3: The Birth of the Prison*. London: Vintage Books.

Fowler, Víctor. 1998. "Homoerotismo y construcción de la nación." *La Gaceta*. 1 (Jan.-Feb.).

Fuentes, Filvio. 1978. "Mohamed Ali con faldas." *Bohemia* 70 (26): 31.

García López-Trigo, Camilo. 2012. "El rumbo ya ha sido trazado, ¡avancemos!" *K1000G*, February 5. Accessed June 22, 2014. http://k1000g.blogspot.co.uk/2012/02/el-rumbo-ya-ha-sido-trazado-avancemos.html.

Gardner, Katy. 1981. "Cuba Focuses on Primary Care." *Medical World* 119 (9–10): 16–18.

Gatell, Jose M. 1989. "Infección por el Virus de la Inmunodeficiencia Humana (HIV)." In *Enfermedades de Transmision Sexual,* edited by Andres Fresnadillo and Rosa M. Humet, 183–88.

Gauri, Varun. 2003. "Social Rights and Economics: Claims to Health Care and Education in Developing Countries." *World Development* 32 (3): 465–77.

Goite Pierre, Mayda. 2013. "Plan de Postgrados 2013." Universdad de la Habana Facultad de Derecho.

Goldberg, Abbie E., Lori A. Kinkler, Hannah B. Richardson and Jordan B. Downing. 2012. "On the Border: Young Adults with LGBQ Parents Navigate LGBTQ Communities." *Journal of Counseling Psychology* 59 (1): 71–85.

González Delgado, Dalia. 2013. "Hogar es amor, respeto e inclusión." *Granma,* May 10. Accessed June 22, 2014. http://www.cenesex.org/2013/05/hogar-es-amor-respeto-e-inclusion/.

González Hernández, C. Alicia and Beatriz Castellanos Simons. 2006. *Sexualidad y Géneros: Alternativas para su educación ante los retos del siglo XXI.* 2nd ed. Havana: Editorial Científico-Técnica.

González Pagés, Julio César. 2010. *Macho varón masculino. Estudios de masculinidades en Cuba.* Havana: Editorial de la Mujer.

———. 2014a. "No a los crímenes de odio en Cuba: asesinato del director de teatro Tony Díaz." *Masculinidades en Cuba,* Janaury 31. Accessed June 22, 2014. http://masculinidadescuba.blogspot.co.uk/2014/01/no-los-crimenes-de-odio-en-cuba.html.

———. 2014b. "Un duro golpe para el teatro cubano y la comunidad LGBT." *Red Observatorio Crítico,* February 1. Accessed June 22, 2014. http://observatoriocriticocuba.org/2014/02/01/asesinan-a-tony-diaz/.

González Plasencia, Yolanda. 1996. "Momentos culminantes del pensamiento de Fidel sobre la mujer cubana." In *La mujer en la Revolución y la Revolución en la mujer,* edited by Carolina Aguilar Ayerra and Isabel Moya, 41–46. Havana: Editorial de la Mujer.

González, Ray. 1996. *Muy macho: Latin men confront their manhood.* New York: Anchor Books.

Gotkowitz, Laura and Turits Richard. 1984. "Fiction or Documentary? Screenwriter Ambrosio Fornet on UMAP and Improper Conduct." *Gay Community News* 12 (11): 9.

Granma. 1972. "En el XII Aniversario de la FMC." August 13.

———. 1977a. "Clausurado el IV Congreso Nacional del sindicato de los trabajadores de la salud." October 14.

———. 1977b. "Sobre el pleno ejercicio de la igualdad de la mujer." September 3.

———. 1977c. "Texto del dictamen de la comisión de atención a la infancia y a la igualdad de derechos de la mujer sobre el proyecto de ley modificativa del Código de Familia." June 15.

Granma Internacional. 2014. "Margaret Chan Impressed by Cuba's Healthcare Achievements." July 16. Accessed August 25, 2015. http://www.granma.cu/idiomas/ingles/cuba-i/16julio-chan-salud.html.

Grogg, Patricia. 2009. "Arranca campaña contra la homofobia en Cuba." *IPS,* March 27. Accessed June 22, 2014. http://www.ipsnoticias.net/2009/03/sociedad-cuba-arranca-campana-contra-la-homofobia/.

Guarnero, Peter A., and Jacquekyn H. Flaskerud. 2014. "Health and Health Research Needs of the LGBTI Community." *Mental Health Nursing* 35 (9): 721–23.

Guevara, Ernesto. 1997. "Speech to Medical Students and Health Workers." In *Che Guevara Reader,* edited by David Deutschman, 112–20. Melbourne: Ocean Press.

Guillard Limonta, Norma. 2009. "Cuba and the Revolutionary Struggle to Transform a Sexist Consciousness: Lesbians on the Cuba Screen." *Latin American Perspectives* 36 (1): 63–71.

Hamilton, Carrie. 2012. *Sexual Revolutions in Cuba.* Chapel Hill: University of North Carolina Press.

Haraway, Donna. 2000. "A Cyborg Manifesto: Science, Technology and Social-Feminism in the Late 20th Century." In *The Cybercultures Reader*, edited by David Bell and Barbara M. Kennedy, 291–315. London: Routledge.

Harman, Sophie. 2012. *Global Health Governance*. New York: Routledge.

Hartmann, Heidi. 1981. "The Unhappy Marriage of Marxist and Feminism: Toward a More Progressive Union." In *Women and Revolution: A Discussion of the Unhappy Marriage of Marxist and Feminism*, edited by Lydia Sargent, 1–42. Montreal: Black Rose Books.

Hernández, Óscar Misael. 2008. "Debates y aportes en los estudios sobre mascilinidades en Méxio." *Relaciones. Estudios de hsitoria y sociedad* 29 (116): 231–53.

Hirai, Michiyo, Mark H. Winkel, and Jason R. Popan. 2014. "The role of machismo in prejudice toward lesbians and gay men: Personality traits as moderators." *Personality and Individual Differences* 70: 105–10.

Hirschfeld, Katherine. 2007. *Health, Politics, and Revolution in Cuba Since 1898*. New Brunswick: Transaction Publishers.

Hoffman, Sarah. 2005. "HIV/AIDS in Cuba: A Model For Care Or An Ethical Dilemma?" *African Health Sciences* 4 (2): 208–9.

Huish, Robert. 2013. *Where No Doctor Has Gone Before*. Waterloo: Wilfrid Laurier University Press.

Ibrahim, Abadir M. 2015. "LGBT rights in Africa and the discursive role of international human rights law." *African Human Rights Law Journal* 15 (2): 263–81.

InfoMed. 2013. "Noticias SEXSALUD 2013." I Cónclave Virtual Nacional de Estudiantes Universitarios en Foro Virtual Sobre Sexualidad. Accessed July 14, 2014. http://promociondeeventos.sld.cu/sexsalud2013/noticias-sexsalud-2013/.

Informe de Cuba en virtud de lo establecido en la resolución 60/224 Titulado. 2006. "Preparativos y organización de la reunión de 2006 dedicada al seguimiento de los resultados del vigésimo sexto período extraordinario de sesiones: Aplicación de la declaración de compromiso en la lucha contra el VIH/SIDA." 14 March.

Iñiguez, Luisa. 2013. "Overview of Evolving Changes in Cuba's Health Services." *MEDICC Review* 15 (2): 45–51.

IPS. 2012a. "Educación sexual por todos los derecho." January 26. Accessed September 20, 2014. http://www.ipscuba.net/index.php?option=com_k2&view=item&id=3118:educaci%C3%B3n-sexual-por-todos-los-derechos&Itemid=5.

———. 2012b. "Programa de la 5ta Jornada contra la homofobia." April 16. Accessed June 22, 2014. http://www.ipscuba.net/index.php?option=com_k2&view=item&id=3936:programa-de-la-5ta-jornada-cubana-contra-la-homofobia&Itemid=5.

———. 2012c. "Proyecto HSH: logros paso a paso." June 1. Accessed June 22, 2014. http://www.ipscuba.net/index.php?option=com_k2&view=item&id=4374:proyecto-hsh-logros-paso-a-paso&Itemid=5.

Jorge. 2009. "Resentado el documental sobre la Jornada Cubana contra la Homofobia 2009." *Red Peruana TLGB*, August 28. Accessed June 22, 2014. http://www.redperuanatlgb.net/index.php?option=com_content&task=view&id=450&Itemid=37.

Juventudrebelde.cu. 2007. "Aumentan hombres que usan atributos femeninos." November 11. Accessed June 22, 2014. http://www.juventudrebelde.cu/cuba/2007-11-11/aumentan-hombres-que-usan-atributos-femeninos/.

Kapcia, Antoni. 2008. *Cuba in revolution: A history since the fifties*. London: Reaktion Books.

———. 2014. *Leadership in the Cuban Revolution: The Unseen Story*. London: Zed Books.

———. 2016. "Interview: Antoni Kapcia." E-International Relations, November 17. Accessed January 8, 2017. http://www.e-ir.info/2016/11/17/interview-antoni-kapcia/

Kinsey, Alfred C., Wardell Baxter Pomeroy, and Clyde Eugene Martin. 1948. *Sexual Behavior in the Human Male*. Bloomington: Indiana University Press.

Kinsey, Alfred C., Wardell Baxter Pomeroy, Clyde Eugene Martin, and Gebhard Paul H. 1953. *Sexual Behavior in the Human Female*. Bloomington: Indiana University Press.

Kirk, Emily J. 2011. "Setting the Agenda for Cuban Sexuality: The Role of Cuba's CENESEX." *Canadian Journal for Latin American Studies* 36 (72): 143–64.

———. 2015. "The Changing Dynamics of Sexuality: CENESEX and the Revolution." In *A Contemporary Cuba Reader: The Revolution under Raúl Castro*, edited by Phillip Brenner, Marguerite Rose Jiménez, John M. Kirk, and William M. Leogrande, 433–40. Lanham: Rowman and Littlefield.

Kirk, John M. and Michael H. Erisman. 2009. *Cuban Medical Internationalism: Origins, Evolution and Goals*. New York: Palgrave Macmillan.

Krause, Monika. 1985. *Algunos temas fundamentales sobre la educación sexual*. Havana: Editorial Científico-Técnica.

———. 1987. *Algunos temas fundamentales sobre la educación sexual*. 2nd Edition. Havana: Editorial Científico-Técnica.

———. 1988. *Educación sexual. Selección de lecturas*. Havana: Editorial Científico-Técnica.

Krause-Fuchs, Monika. 2007. *¿Machismo? No gracias. Cuba: sexualidad en la revolución*. Santa Cruz de Tenerife: Ediciones Ideal.

Labacena Romero, Yuniel and Katheryn Felipe González. 2011. "Todo el mundo cuenta." *Juventud Rebelde*, April 13. Accessed June 22, 2014. http://www.juventudrebelde.cu/suplementos/sexo-sentido/2011-04-22/todo-el-mundo-cuenta/.

Larguía, Isabel. 1973. "The Economic Basis of the Status of Women." Paper presented at the IX International Congress of Anthropological and Ethnological Sciences, University of Warwick Communist Party, Coventry.

La República. 2012. "Anuncian estudio acerca de represión contra homosexuales en Cuba." April 13. Accessed September 20, 2014. http://www.larepublica.pe/23-04-2012/anuncian-estudio-acerca-de-represion-contra-homosexuales-en-Cuba.

La Rose, Lauren. 2016. "Q&A: George Takei on Canada as an LGBT rights leader and meeting with PM Trudeau." *The Canadian Press*, May 21. Accessed January 8, 2017. http://thechronicleherald.ca/artslife/1366399-qa-george-takei-on-canada-as-an-lgbt-rights-leader-and-meeting-with-pm-trudeau.

Lavrin, Asunción. 1998. "International Feminisms: Latin American Alternatives." *Gender and History* 10 (3): 519–34.

LeBreton, Artidoro Cáceres. 1997. "Homosexualidad ego-distónica." *Sexología y Sociedad* 3 (7): 15–19.

Leiner, Marvin. 1994. *Sexual Politics in Cuba: Machismo, Homosexuality and AIDS*. Boulder: Westview Press.

Leyva, Anneris and Iris de Armas. 2010. "Sexualidad, educación y salud como bases de un mundo mejor." *Granma*, January 20.

Lockwood, Lee. 1967. *Castro's Cuba, Cuba's Fidel*. New York: Vintage Books.

López, Cory. 2007. "Especialista cubana llama al respeto a las preferencias sexuales." World Data Service, May 21. Accessed May 19, 2012. http://www.profesionalespcm.org/_php/MuestraArticulo2.php?id=8718.

López Nodarse, Mérida M. 1994. "La investigación: Una de las líneas de trabajo de Centro Nacional de Educación Sexual." *Sexología y Sociedad* 1 (0): 32–33.

Lumsden, Ian. 1996. *Machos, Maricones and Gays: Cuba and Homosexuality*. Philadelphia: Temple University Press.

Lutjens, Sheryl L. 1995. "Reading between the lines: Women, the state, and rectification in Cuba." *Latin American Perspectives* 22 (2): 100–24.

MacDonald, Théodore. 1993. *Hippocrates in Havana. Cuba's Health Care System*. Mexico City: Bolivar Books.

Macmillan S., Guillermo and Perla Yunge Ducaud. 2002. "Experiencia Quirúrgica en transexualismo de psiquis femenina." *Sexología y Sociedad* 8 (18): 12–14.

Madero, Abel Sierra. 2016. "Lo de las UMAP fue un trabajo 'top secret': Entrevista a la Dra. María Elena Solé Arrondo." *Cuban Studies* 44: 357–66.

Maderos Machado, María. 1994. "La educación en la población desde la educación de la sexualidad en la escuela cubana." *Sexología y Sociedad* 1 (0): 16–17.

Marilley, Suzan M. 1996. *Women Suffrage and the Origins of Liberal Feminism in the United States 1820-1920*. Cambridge: Harvard University Press.

Masters, William and Virginia E. Johnson. 1966. *Human Sexual Response*. Boston: Little, Brown & Co.

Matos, Orlando. 2006. "Cuba: Not Everyone Ready for Prime Time TV AIDS Story." *IPS*, June 19. Accessed June 22, 2014. https://groups.yahoo.com/neo/groups/CubaVerdad/conversations/messages/23658.

Maynard, Steven. 2002. "Gays and the Cuban revolution: The case of Reinaldo Arenas." *Latin American Perspectives* 29 (2): 78–98.

McPherson Sayú, Margarita. 1995. "El Maestro: Agente de cambio." *Sexología y Sociedad* 1 (2): 7–9.

MEDICC Review. 2013. "Primary Health Care: Starting Point for Health Equity." 15 (2): 3.

Menéndez Dávila, Mileyda. 2011. "Jornada por el Día Mundial de la Salud Sexual." *Juventud Rebelde*, September 1. Accessed May 19, 2011. http://www.juventudrebelde.cu/cuba/2011-09-01/jornada-por-el-dia-mundial-de-la-salud-sexual/.

Menéndez Dávila, Mileyda and Omar Parada. 2010. "Hermes Despeja interrogantes." *Juventud Rebelde*, March 5. Accessed June 22, 2014. http://www.juventudrebelde.cu/suplementos/sexo-sentido/2010-03-05/hermes-despeja-interrogantes/.

MINED. 1981. *Ministerio de Educación, Instituto Central de Ciencias Pedagogias Informe sobre la investigación: Perfeccionamiento de los métodos y formas organizativas de la educación sexual en el proceso docente-educativo*. Havana.

Mirandé, Alfredo. 1997. *Hombres y machos: masculinity and Latino culture*. Boulder: Westview Press.

Mohanty, Chandra Talpade. 1991. "Under Western Eyes: Feminist Scholarship and Colonial Discourses." In *Third World Women and The Politics of Feminism*, edited by Chandra Talpade Mohanty, Ann Russo, and Lourdes Torres, 51–80. Bloomington: Indiana University Press.

Montero Maldonado, Elsa. 1996. "'El pelotón' Mariana Granjales": Expresión de la concepción de Fidel sobre el papel de la mujer en la lucha revolucionaria." In *La Mujer en la Revolución y la Revolución en la mujer*, edited by Carolina Aguilar Ayerra and Isabel Moya, 33–36. Havana: Editorial de la Mujer.

Morales Rodríguez, Giselle. 2013. "Del lobo y el bosque, al hombre nuevo." *Escambray*, June 29.

Morales Suárez, Ileana del Rosario, José A. Fernández Sacasas, and Francisco Durán García. 2008. "Cuban Medical Education: Aiming for Six-Star Doctor." *MEDICC Review* 10 (4): 5–9.

Navarro, V. 1972. "Report of Health Services in Cuba: Health, Health Services, and Health Planning in Cuba." *International Journal of Health Services* 2 (3): 397–432.

Narayan, Uma. 1997. *Dislocating Cultures: Identities, Traditions and Third-World Feminism*. London: Routledge.

Neusy, André-Jacques and Bjorg Plasdottir. 2008. "A Roundtable of Innovative Leaders in Medical Education." *MEDICC Review* 10 (4): 20–24.

Norandi, Mariana. 2009. "En Cuba el cambio de sexo es un servicio gratuito: Mariela Castro." *La Jornada*, September 29. Accessed July 22, 2014. http://www.jornada.unam.mx/2009/09/29/index.php?section=ciencias&article=a02n1cie.

No transfobia. Editorial CENESEX, UNDP, and El fundo mundial de lucha contra el SIDA, la tuberculosis y la malaria. Pamphlet.

Nova, Guillermo. 2010. "Mariela Castro: Ver los prejuicios nos permite trabajar con ellos." *Cubadebate*, February 4. Accessed September 20, 2013. http://www.cubadebate.cu/noticias/2010/02/04/mariela-castro-prejuicios-nos-permite-trabajar-ellos/#.U2ewpceTY7A.

Ocasio, Rafael. 2002. "Gays and the Cuban Revolution: The Case of Reinaldo Arenas." *Latin American Perspectives* 29 (2): 78–98.

Ortega Guzmán, Edimirta 1996. "Las Marianas del Moncada." In *La Mujer en la Revolución y la Revolución en la mujer*, edited by Carolina Aguilar Ayerra and Isabel Moya, 29–32. Havana: Editorial de la Mujer.

Oxfam International. 2008. *Cuba's HIV/AIDS Strategy: An Integrated, Rights-Based Approach*. Oxfam.

Padrón Durán, Rubén S. 2006. "Las hormonas y su relación con transexualidad." *Sexología y Sociedad* 12 (31): 11–19.

Pantaleón, Doris. 2009. "Hija de Raúl Castro dice sólo educación sexual logrará cambio conducta para frenar sida." *Listin Diario*, September 15. Accessed June 22, 2014. http://listindiario.com.do/la-republica/2009/9/15/114954/print-no-pics.

Paquito. 2013. "El nuevo Código de Trabajo podría proteger por primera vez los derechos de los homosexuales." *Rebelión*, August 30. Accessed June 22, 2014. http://paquitoeldecuba.com/2013/08/02/nuevo-codigo-de-trabajo-podria-proteger-por-primera-vez-derechos-de-homosexuales-en-cuba/.

PCC. 1976. *Sobre el pleno ejercicio de la igualdad de la mujer. Tesis y resolución*. Havana: Departamento de Orientación Revolucionaria del Comité del Partido Comunista de Cuba.

———. 1980a. *Proyecto de Resoluciones sobre las Tesis aprobadas por el I Congreso del Partido Comunista de Cuba*. Havana: Grupo de publicaciones II Congreso del Partido Comunista de Cuba, Editorial Política.

———. 1980b. *Segundo Congreso del Partido Comunista de Cuba. Proyecto de Resoluciones sobre las Tesis aprobadas por el I Congreso del Partido Comunista de Cuba*. Havana: Departamento de Orientación Revolucionaria del Comité del Partido Comunista de Cuba.

———. 2016. "7mo Congreso PCC. Conceptualización del modelo económico y social cubano de desarrollo socialista." Accessed March 20, 2016. http://www.cubadebate.cu/wp-content/uploads/2016/05/Copia-para-el-Sitio-Web.pdf.

Peláez, Jorge and Aldo Rodríguez. 1996. "Aborto en la adolescencia." *Sexología y Sociedad* 2 (5): 2–5.

Peña, Manuel. 1991. "Class, gender and machismo: The 'treacherous-woman' folklore of Mexican male workers." *Gender and Society* 5 (1): 30–46.

Peña, Susana. 2007. "'Obvious Gay' and the State Gaze: Cuban Gay Visibility and U.S. Immigration Policy during the 180 Mariel Boatlift." *Journal of the History of Sexuality* 16 (3): 482–514.

Pérez, Christina. 2008. *Caring for Them from Birth to Death: The Practice of Community-Based Cuban Medicine.* Lanham: Lexington Books.

Pérez, Evelio J., Alpizar María E., Cobas Cobiella, and Mercedes Rodríguez Acosta. 2002. "Legal and Ethical Aspects of HIV/AIDS in Cuba." *MEDICC Review.* Accessed July 2, 2012. http://www.medicc.org/publications/medicc_review/III/hiv-aids/pages/legal.html.

Pérez, Jorge, Daniel Pérez, Ida Gonzales, Manuel Diaz Jidy, Mylai Orta, Carlos Aragonés, José Joanes, Manuel Santín, Maria Isela Lantero, Rigoberta Torres, Ailen González, and Alejandro Álvarez. 2004. "Approaches to the Management of HIV/AIDS in Cuba." *World Health Organization*. Geneva.

Pineda Barnet, Enrique. 2012. "Estrenará el Cineclub Diferente la película cubana 'Verde Verde'." *Puentear*, February 7. Accessed June 22, 2014. http://puentear.blogspot.co.uk/2012/02/estrenara-el-cineclub-diferente-la.html.

Powell, Colin L. 2004. "Commission for assistance to a free Cuba. Report to the president." Washington, DC, U.S. Department of State. Accessed September 21, 2013. http://pdf.usaid.gov/pdf_docs/PCAAB192.pdf.

Prendes Labrada, Marianela de la C., and Wilfredo Guibert Reyes. 2007. *Adolescente embarazada: ¿La mejor opción?*. Havana: Editorial Científico-Técnica.

Prensa Latina. 2014. "Realizarán en Cuba VII Jornada contra la Homofobia." April 23. Accessed April 23, 2014. http://www.prensa-latina.cu/index.php?option=com_content&task=view&id=2609541&Itemid=1.

Prieto Morales, Abel. 1969. "Homosexualismo." *Bohemia* 61 (8): 108-113.

Progreso Semanal, Aurelio Pedroso. 2012. "De Travesti a Concejal." *Rebelión*, November, 19. Accessed June 22, 2014. http://www.rebelion.org/noticia.php?id=159404.

Proveyer Cervantes, Clotilde, Reina Fleites Ruiz, Graciela González Olmedo, Blanca Múster Infante, and María Auxiliadora César. 2011. *50 years later: Women and social change in Cuba*. Edited by Mana M. Diaz, translated by Jesse Kates-Chinoy and Emily Carpenter. Havana: Oxfam.

Puentes, Lisandra. 2012. "Cine Club Diferente: desterrando prejuicios." *Tribuna de la Habana*, May 14. Accessed June 22, 2014. http://www.tribuna.co.cu/cultura/2012-05-14/cine-club-diferente-desterrando-prejuicios.

Puentes Valladares, Lisandra. 2013a. "Cónclave santiaguero para toda la Isla." CENESEX. Accessed June 22, 2014. http://www.cenesex.org/2013/01/conclave-santiaguero-para-toda-la-isla/.

Quintana Llanio, Livia. *Maternidad, paternidad y familia. Con enfoque de género y derechos.* Promoción y Comercio del Caribe. Pamphlet.

Quiroga, José. 2000. *Tropics of Desire: Interventions from Queer Latino America*. New York: New York University Press.

Ramírez, Marta María. 2013. Interview with Emily J. Kirk. February 4. Havana.

Randall, Margaret. 1974. *Cuban Women Now: Afterword 1974*. Toronto: The Women's Press.

———. 1978. *No se puede hacer la revolución sin nosotras*. Havana: Ediciones Casa de las Américas.

———. 1981. *Women in Cuba*. New York: Smyrna Press.

———. 1992. *Gathering Rage: The Failure of 20th Century Revolutions to Develop a Feminist Agenda*. New York: Monthly Review Press.

Rawls, John. 1971. *A Theory of Justice*. Cambridge: Harvard University Press.

Ravelo, Ayolma. 1989. *Del amor, hablemos francamente*. Havana: Editorial Gente Nueva.

———. 1999. "Hablemos francamente: De ti también depende mujer que el SIDA no decide." *Mujeres* 1: 12–13.

———. 2002. "Hablemos francamente: Esa manera de amar." *Mujeres* 4: 64–66.

———. 2005. *Intimidades: Adolescencia y Sexualidad*. Havana: Editorial Científico-Técnica, Instituto Cubano del Libro.

———. 2007a. "Hablemos francamente: Andopausia ¿Qué pasa con el hombre que envejece?" *Mujeres* 2: 82–84.

———. 2007b. "Hablemos francamente: Intimidad matrimonial." *Mujeres* 1: 82–84.

———. 2008. *Enigmas de la sexualidad femenina*. 2nd ed. Havana: Federación de Mujeres Cubanas, Editorial de la Mujer.

———. 2009. *40 preguntas sobre sexo*. Havana: Editorial Mujeres Cubanas, Editorial de la Mujer.

———. 2011. *Sexo, amor y erotismo*. Havana: Editorial de la Mujer.

Reed, Gail A. 2006. "HIV in Cuba: Prevention of Mother-to-Child Transmission." *Medicc Review* 8 (1). Accessed June 22, 2014. http://www.medicc.org/publications/medicc_review/0406/mr-interview.html.

Reuters. 2010. "Fidel Castro Takes Blame for 1960s Gay Persecution." August 31. Accessed November 1, 2011. http://www.reuters.com/article/2010/08/31/us-Cuba-castro-idUSTRE67U4JE20100831.

Ring, Jennifer. 1985. "Mill's The Subjection of Women: The Methodological Limits of Liberal Feminism." *The Review of Politics* 47 (1): 27–44.

Ring, Trudy. 2013. "Mariela Castro Points to Progress on LGBT Rights in Cuba." *The Advocate*, May 5. Accessed September 20, 2014. http://www.advocate.com/politics/2013/05/05/mariela-castro-points-progress-lgbt-rights-Cuba.

Rivero Pino, Ramón, ed. 2014. *Lo local-comunitario*. Havana: Editorial CENESEX.

Roca Perara, Miguel Angel. 2011. *Los jóvenes preguntan acerca de la pareja*. Havana: Instituto Cubano del Libro, Ediciones Libre.

Rodríguez, Andrea. 2012. "Transgender woman 1st to win office in Cuba." *Associated Press*, November 12. Accessed June 22, 2014. http://www.thejakartapost.com/news/2012/11/17/transgender-woman-1st-win-office-cuba.html.

Rodríguez Boti, Regino. 2003. *La sexualidad al atardecer de la vida*. Santiago de Cuba: Instituto Cubano del Libro, Editorial del Oriente.

Rodríguez Lauzurique, Mayra. 1994. "Formación de promotores juveniles." *Sexología y Sociedad* 1 (0): 30–31.

Rodríguez Lauzurique, Rosa Mayra. 2005. *Prevenir desde la diversidad sexual. Programa para la formación de promotores en salud sexual con enfasis en ITS-VIH/SIDA en hombres travestis que tienen sexo con otros hombres (travestis/HSH)*. Havana: Editorial CENESEX.

———. 2013. Interview with Emily J. Kirk. February 20. Havana.

Rodríguez Lauzurique, Rosa Mayra, Ada C. Alfonso Rodríguez, and Magaly González Jiménez. 2009. *Prevenir desde la diversidad sexual. Herramientas para el autocuidado y la prevención de las ITS y el VIH*. Havana: Editorial CENESEX.

Rojas Ochoa, Francisco. 2003. "La enseñanza de la salud pública a estudiantes de medicina." *Revista Cubana Educación Médica Superior* 17 (2). Accessed August 22, 2014. http://www.bvs.sld.cu/revistas/ems/vol17_2_03/ems01203.htm.

Roque Guerra, Alberto. 2009. "Diversidad sexual en Cuba, ¿Cortina de humo o miopía académica?" *Rebelión*, August 12. Accessed June 22. http://www.rebelion.org/noticia.php?id=89957.

———. 2011. "Sexual Diversity in Revolutionary Times, 1959–2009." *Cuban Studies* 42: 218–26.

———. 2013a. "Carta Abierta al Presidente del Parlamento cubano, compañero Esteban Lazo, sobre Anteproyecto de Ley Código de Trabajo." *HOMOsapiens@Cuba*, August 10. Accessed June 22, 2014. http://aroqueg.blogspot.co.uk/2013/08/carta-abierta-al-presidente-del.html.

———. 2013b. "Ciudadanía sexual, participación y emancipación: antecedentes y futuro en Cuba." *IPS*, July 13. Accessed June 22, 2014. http://www.ipscuba.net/index.php?option=com_k2&view=item&id=7662:ciudadan%C3%ADa-sexual-participación-y-emancipación-antecedentes-y-futuro-en-cuba&Itemid=5.

Rosales, Anna. 2012. "Cubanos contra la homofobia." *Radio Nederland*, May 17. Accessed September 20, 2014. http://archief.rnw.nl/espanol/article/cubanos-contra-la-homofobia.

Rowe, Michael. 2009. "New Cuban Revolution?" *The Advocate*, September 14. Accessed September 20, 2009. http://www.advocate.com/news/world-news/2009/09/14/new-cuban-revolucion?page=full.

Sahar, Amer. 2012. "Naming to Empower: Lesbianism in the Arab Islamicate World Today." *Journal of Lesbian Studies* 16 (4): 381–97.

Salva, Janet. 1979a. "Y la mujer se ciñó el glorioso uniforme." *Bohemia* 71 (41): 32–37.

———. 1979b. "Una nueva tarea para las mujeres. El III Congreso de su organización." *Bohemia* 70 (6): 6–7.

———. 1979c. "III Congreso de la FMC." *Bohemia* 71 (20): 49.

———. 1980. "La mujer y su papel en la sociedad. Entrevista con Vilma Espín." *Behemia* 72 (10): 50–55.

Salva, Janet, Susana Tesoro, and Manuel González Bello. 1980. "III Congreso de la FMC." *Bohemia* 72 (11): 42–49.

Sandoval, Chela. 1991. "U.S. Third World Feminism: The Theory and Method of Oppositional Consciousness in the Postmodern World." *Gender* 10: 1–24.

San Francisco Chronicle. 2012. "Cuba's Mariela Castro cheered in S.F. visit." May 14. Accessed September 20, 2012. http://www.sfgate.com/cgibin/article.cgi?f=/c/a/2012/05/23/BAFG1OMOLS.DTL.

Santana, Arelys. 2013. "Nuestra revolución: ni colco ni copia." In *Mujeres y Revolución: El ejemplo vivo de la Revolución cubana*, edited by Asela de los Santos, Mary-Alice Waters, Arelys Santana and Leira Sánchez, 11–17. New York: Pathfinder.

Schnabl, Siegfried. 1989. *El hombre y la mujer en la intimidad*. 2nd ed. Havana: Editorial Científico-Técnica.

———. 1981. *En Defensa del Amor*. 2nd ed. Havana: Editorial Científico-Técnica. Seidler, Victor J. 1989. *Rediscovering masculinity: Reason, language and sexuality*. New York: Routledge.

Serrano Lorenzo, Yanesy de la Caridad. 2012. "Conformación de un modelo de masculinidad hegemónica durante la etapa colonial en Cuba." *Sexología y Sociedad* 18 (48): 11–18.

Sierra Madero, Abel. 2003. "La policía del sexo: La homofobia durante el siglo XIX en Cuba." *Sexología y Sociedad* 9 (21): 12–14.

Sierra, Raquel. 2008. "Diversidad sexual: abriendo paso a la comprensión." *Cultura y Sociedad*. No. 1 (January).

Smith, Adam. 1776. *Wealth of Nations. Vol. 2 Book 5*. Edited by R. H. Campbell and A. S. Skinner. Oxford: Clarendon Press.

Smith, Lois M. 1992. "Sexuality and Socialism in Cuba." In *Cuba in Transition: Crisis and Transformation*, edited by Sandor Halebsky and John Kirk, 177–93. Boulder: Westview Press Inc.

Smith, Lois M. and Alfred Padula. 1996. *Sex and Revolution: Women in socialist Cuba*. Oxford: Oxford University Press.

Sosa Marín, Miguel R. 1994. "Derechos reproductivos, salud sexual y reproductiva y planificación familiar." *Sexología y Sociedad* 1 (0): 10–11.

Sotolongo Carrington, Dulce María. 2011. *Nosotras dos. Antología homorótica femenina*. Havana: Ediciones UNIÓN.

Stout, Noelle. 2014. *After Love: Queer Intimacy and Erotic Economies in Post-Soviet Cuba*. Durham: Duke University Press.

Sternberg, Peter. 2000. "Challenging machismo: Promoting sexual and reproductive health with Nicaraguan men." *Gender and Development* 8 (1): 89–99.

Swissinfo. 2010. "Cuba, una Revolución en marcha." September 4. Accessed September 20, 2014. http://www.swissinfo.ch/spa/cuba--una-revolución-en-marcha/28267620.

Sydney Morning Herald. 2012. "Cuba winning AIDS fight as homophobia gives way to tolerance." May 13. Accessed September 20, 2014. http://www.smh.com.au/world/cuba-winning-aids-fight-as-homophobia-gives-way-to-tolerance-20120513-1ykov.html.

TeleSur. 2016. "Cuba: This Lesbian Hip Hop Duo is Fighting Homophobia." March 17. Accessed April 20. http://www.telesurtv.net/english/news/Cuba-This-Lesbian-Hip-Hop-Duo-is-Fighting-Homophobia--20160317-0001.html.

Terra Perú. 2011. "Comunistas Cuba habrían abordado derechos gay." May 11. Accessed September 20, 2014. http://noticias.terra.com.pe/internacional/latinoamerica/comunistas-cuba-habrian-abordado-derechos-gay,08fd97d0c20ef210VgnVCM10000098f154d0RCRD.html.

Terre Morell, Clabriel. 1994. "No me interesa escandalizar: El Diego de *Fresa y chocolate* confiesa que siempre está acelerado." *Bohemia* 86 (8): 4–6.

Thomas, Susan. 2006. "Did Nobody Pass the Girls the Guitars? Queer Appropriations in Contemporary Cuban Popular Song." *Journal of Popular Music Studies* 18 (2): 124–43.

Torres Rodíguez, Beatriz. 2006. *Hablemos de sexualidad. Inquietudes más frecuentes sobre la sexualidad, el amor y la pareja*. Havana: Editorial Científico-Técnica.

———. 2008. *La sexualidad en la adolescencia: ¿Amiga o enemiga?* Havana: Editorial Científico-Técnica.

"Tu condición de mujer." CENESEX, MINSAP, UNDP, El Fundo Mundial de lucha contra el SIDA, la tuberculosis y la malaria. Pamphlet.

Turner, Dwayne C. 1989. "The Homosexual Sons and Daughters of the Cuban Revolution: Steps to Liberation." *Human Mosaic* 23: 60–78.

UNAIDS. 2012. "The Status of HIV in the Caribbean." Accessed July 8, 2016. http://www.unaids.org/en/media/unaids/contentassets/documents/countryreport/2010/2010_HIVInCaribbean_en.pdf.

UNESCO. 1971. "XXXIII Conferencia Internacional de Educación OIE-UNESCO, 15–23 Septiembre." Informe de Cuba. Organización de Educación (UN. Doc. OIE/Q/70/3).

Accessed October 20, 2014. http://www.ibe.unesco.org/National_Reports/Cuba/nr_mf_cu_1971_sef.pdf.

UN News. 2014. "In Cuba, Ban spotlights sustainable development, human rights, gender-based violence." January 28. Accessed September 20, 2014. http://www.un.org/apps/news/story.asp?NewsID=47023.

Valdés Stable, Marcelino. 1977. "Los 'derechos' de la mujer norteamericana." *Granma*. June 14.

Valle Artiz, Pedro Pablo. 2013. Interview with Emily J. Kirk. January 29. Havana.

Vázquez Seijido, Manuel. 2013. Interview with Emily J. Kirk. February 13. Havana.

———. 2014. "Derechos sexuales relativos a la orientación sexual y la identidad de género: algunas reflexiones sobre sus garantías." Paper presented at the annual Latin American Studies Association Congress, Chicago, Illinois, May 21–24.

WebCENESEX, email message to author, June 8, 2012a. "Cineclub 'Diferente' de junio, con filme británico 'Maurice.'"

———. email message to author, May 5, 2012b. "Retrospectiva del cineclub Diferente durante la 5ta Jornada Cubana contra la Homofobia."

Wendell, Susan. 1987. "A (Qualified) Defense of Liberal Feminism." *Hypathia* 2 (2): 65–93.

What's on Havana! 2014. Accessed May 20, 2014. http://www.cubaabsolutely.com/What's-On-Havana-May-2014.pdf.

Whiteford, Linda M. and Laurence G. Branch. 2008. *Primary Health Care in Cuba: The Other Revolution*. Plymouth: Rowman & Littlefield Publishers.

Whitehead, Stephen M. 2002. *Men and Masculinities*. Cambridge: Polity Press.

Wiseman, John and Kathleen Brasher. 2008. "Community Wellbeing in an Unwell World: Trends, Challenges, and Possibilities." *Journal of Public Health Policy* 29 (3): 353–66.

Yglesias, José. 1968. *In the Fist of the Revolution*. New York: Pantheon Books.

Index

About the Author

Emily J. Kirk is a Social Sciences and Humanities Research Council (SSHRC) Postdoctoral Research Fellow in the Department of International Development Studies at Dalhousie University. She received her MPhil from the University of Cambridge and her PhD from the University of Nottingham. Her research interests focus on global health, Latin American development issues, and south-south cooperation. Much of her work focuses on Cuba, where she has carried out extensive research, and she is currently writing about different aspects of the Cuban development model.

www.ingramcontent.com/pod-product-compliance
Lightning Source LLC
LaVergne TN
LVHW101448200926
848483LV00001B/90
* 9 7 8 1 4 9 8 5 5 7 6 6 5 *